Sensory Wellness

THE ART AND SCIENCE OF THRIVING

Robyn Chu MOT, OTR/L

SENSORY WELLNESS
THE ART AND SCIENCE OF THRIVING

All marketing and publishing rights guaranteed to and reserved by:

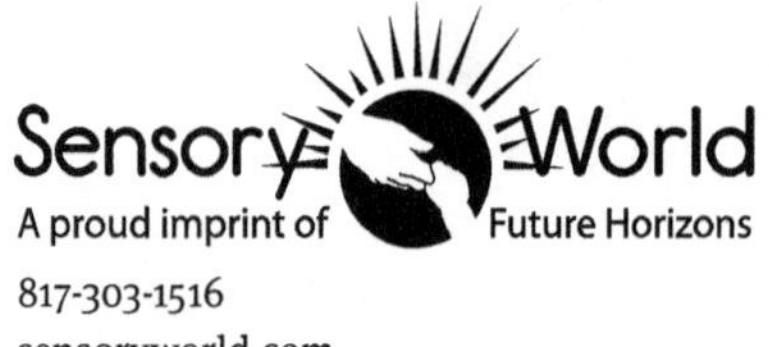

817-303-1516
sensoryworld.com

Illustrated by Samantha LeDuc

ISBN: 978-1-963367-54-6

DEDICATION

This book is dedicated to my children.
You inspire me to live fully, love deeply, and blossom
in ways I never imagined possible.
I love you all more than words can express!

TABLE OF CONTENTS

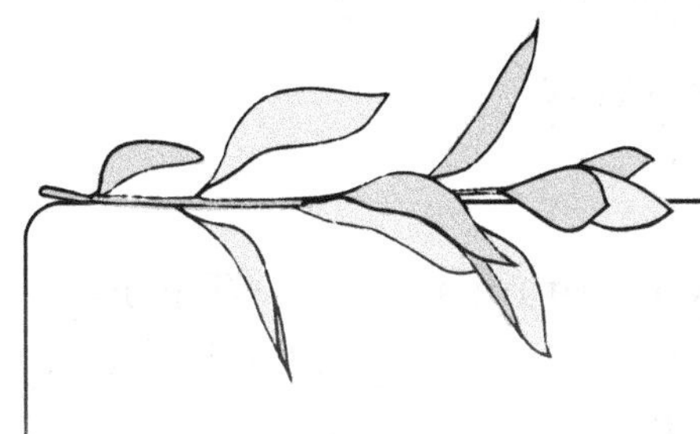

AUTHOR'S NOTE

"Truth like infinity is to be forever approached but never reached."

- A. Jean Ayres, PhD, OTR -

This world is experiencing an unprecedented information overload with the explosion of podcasts, videos online, and websites about almost any topic you can imagine. I didn't want to add to the noise by writing a book that contributed to this information overload. While this book *is* informational, I wrote with the intent of giving you an eye-opening, expanding-your-possibilities way of thinking about sensory health. I hope this book is not only informative but also experiential for you: a fork in the road of the journey of your life. Sensory wellness can breathe life into the darkest corners of your being, creating choices when you could only see one way and increasing your agency to make the changes you want to be your best self. I invite you into *Sensory Wellness* as the beginning of a mind-body integrative experience.

The reflection questions and sensory exploration exercises throughout this book will guide you along your journey, deepening your friendship with your brain and body. Through this interactive experience, I hope you and all people feel welcome, included, worthy, celebrated, seen, and heard. I invite you to use the elements of sensation, like paint and brushes for an artist, to create a masterpiece of sensory wellness in your life!

This book is the combined effort of my own personal journey as a woman, daughter, sister, friend, wife, and mother, and my professional voyage as an occupational therapist. I personally have done this work and have been honored to walk beside many clients, families, and other helping professionals on their journeys. Stories throughout this book are real and sometimes have been adapted to support the anonymity of the people whose stories are being told. The people I have journeyed with both clinically and personally are diverse in neurodevelopmental process, age, race, ethnicity, socioeconomic status, marital status, educational attainment, employment, religion, gender identity, and geographic location. While I am deeply committed to learning and sharing in a way that honors each person I have had the privilege of connecting with, I acknowledge the limitations of my experiences and racial and economic privilege in bringing you the information and exploration activities in this book. I look forward to learning more in the journey ahead and, as Maya Angelo invites: doing better when I know better.

The journey of writing this book has been a wonderful learning process, one I am committed to continuing. Implementing what I have learned has helped me and the people I love. I hope the sensory wellness movement contributes to a more just and loving world. Onward, ever present.

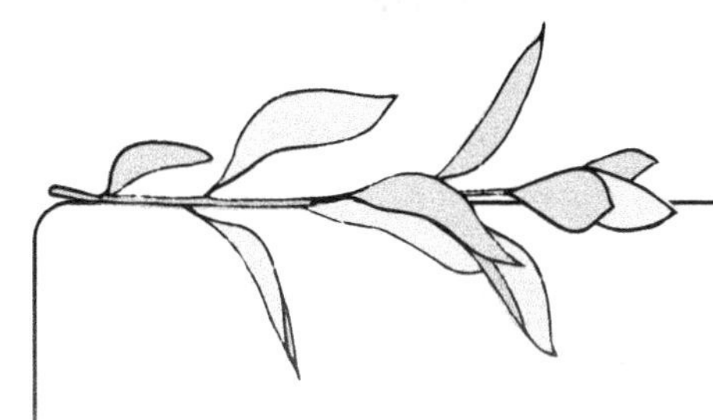

WITH GRATITUDE

This book is both the culmination and the beginning, thanks to so many.

To God: I hope this book conveys the light and blessing You whispered into my heart. Thank You for Your love, Your guidance, and the never-ending piggyback ride that is the wild and exciting journey of life.

To my parents, Peanut and Tena Harms: As a parent now, I think back to my early childhood and the messages you received about my physical development and learning differences. I pause with even more awe for the way you responded and guided me every step of the way. When I bristled at your loving embrace, you found other ways to love me well. Thank you for believing in me and opening doors of opportunity. I'm so grateful for the love you showed me, the passionate living you modeled, and the ever-present message that all things are possible.

To my sisters, Christine, Lillian, and Cora: Oh, the sensational quests we created and played! The seeds for this book were planted throughout our childhood as we journeyed to far-off places and different centuries with our imagination while time stood still. You are the best friends and partners in play I could ever hope for! Thank you for always showing up with a shoulder to cry on and a really long hug.

To my extended family: In the most expansive use of the term, thank you for loving me into the person I am today. Through fun adventures and hard seasons, celebrations and mourning, we journey together, and I am better for it. I love you all.

To my beloved friend Jenae Cooper: In all seasons, you ground me, encourage me, and show me God's love. We slowly strolled down the sleepless path of parenting young children, in awe of their wonder and joy. I love diving deep into the research on a variety of topics while simultaneously getting in a workout and running hard toward cheering on our families with full abandon. I'm blessed to do life by your side.

To my mentors, Lucy Jane Miller, PhD, OTR; Elysa Marco, MD; Pratik Mukherjee, MD, PhD; Carol Stock Kranowitz, MA; and Sarah Schoen, PhD, OTR: Thank you for all the ways you helped lay the foundation for this book. Your research, encouragement, guidance, and questions have shaped me and this book. Carol, thank you for your editorial insights! I felt your hugs, nurturing advice, and wisdom as we laughed together, separated only in geographic distance. Working on various projects with each of you over the years has taught me so much, and our friendships are sunshine for my soul. The joy of increasing awareness about sensory integration and processing together has been and will continue to be my calling.

To my co-laboring sensational occupational therapists, Carrie Schmitt, Michele Parkins, Lisa Porter, Renee Allen, Colleen Whiting, Mim Ochsenbein, Gabrielle Perelmuter, and Carolyn Stallings: From graduate school, to creating clinics, to teaching on the STAR faculty, I love our journeys together. It is an honor to create ripples of love and hope with each of you! Carrie, our friendship and Introspection & Interoception adventures have guided so much of my healing, while shaping my heart with your always and forever love. Michele, we will carry the work forward with your light in our hearts and your laughter in our play.

To the Growing Healthy Seasons team (past, present, and future): Thank you all deeply and fully with all my being. Each of you and our work together have helped this book come to be. The amazing directors, Kristi Vecellio, Sandy Chiea, Tena Harms, and Jenni Stucki, show endless love and kindness in supporting our team and many circles of schools and organizations beyond. Our clinical excellence leaders and mentors, Sheryl Trainor, Kara Chapman, Denise Larkin Covello, Angie VanVleet, Amanda Hadley Harriss, Priya Talreja, Casey DeLang, and Emily Finn, encourage learning and growth in their dedication to providing evidence-based, sensory-informed, and play-based therapy for all. And all our inspirational therapists, administrative support team, and developmental specialists are the hands of love, welcoming, encouraging, and passionately serving. Oh, the joy to be in your midst and get to call it work!

To my clients and everyone who gave their stories for this book: This journey would not be the same without each and every one of you. Thank you for teaching me and helping me grow. I am humbled to walk with you.

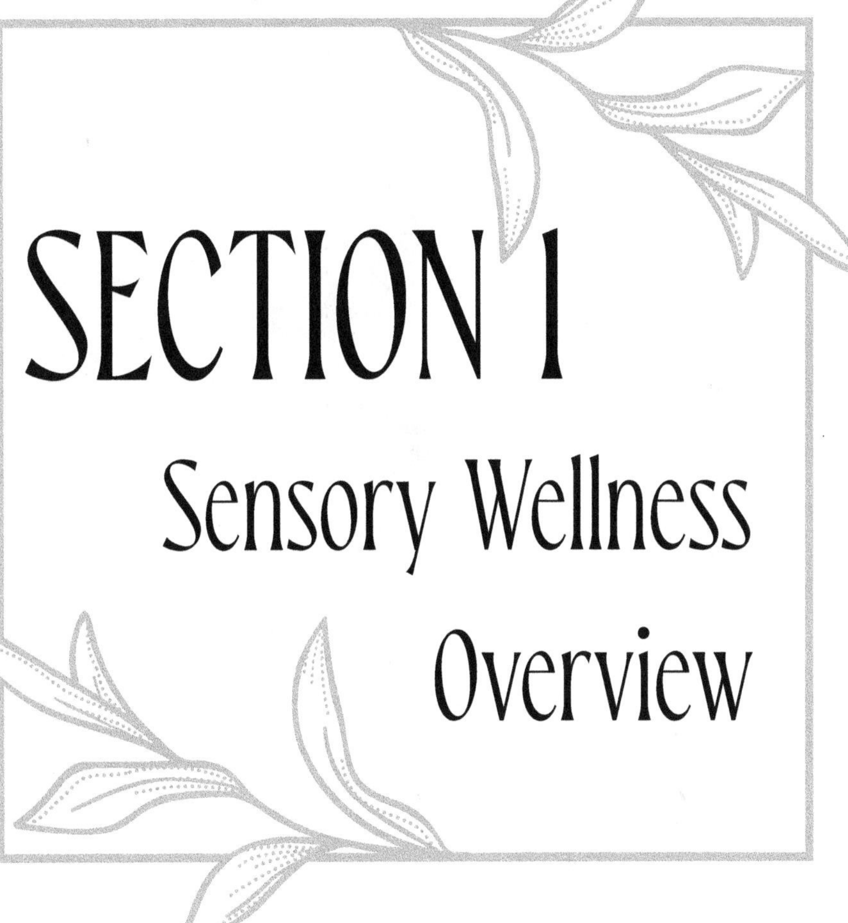

SECTION 1

Sensory Wellness Overview

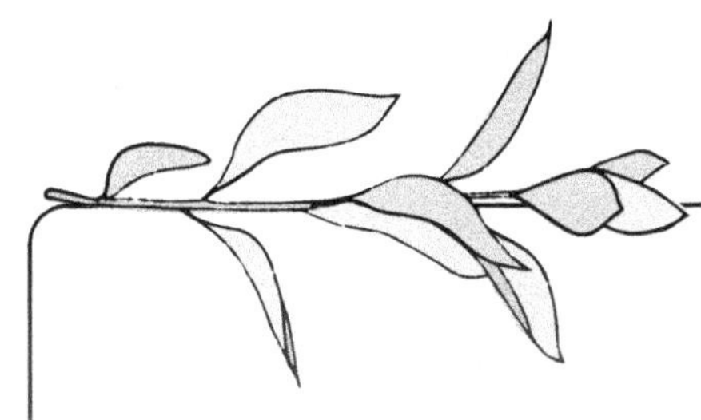

INTRODUCTION

"Sensation is nourishment for the brain."

- A. Jean Ayres, PhD, OTR -

I got an email one day, thought it was a mass marketing message, and moved to the next one, quickly trying to get through the barrage of morning emails that was my daily norm. But something about it stuck. Its words, "My leadership team has all the training on time management and so many leadership techniques. They know their areas of expertise so well ... and yet ..." circled around my head for the next couple of days, and, "My team wants support with the skills underneath these trainings ..." danced through my soul.

Something about this particular "ask" stuck, so I replied to the email: "I appreciate your email, but I think you sent it by mistake. If you could take me off the mass email list, that would be great. I'm already a customer, and I appreciate what you guys do so much!"

But it wasn't a mass email, and I am so grateful the sender responded with grace and love. You see, this "mass email"–sending business owner knew about the work I do with people whose sensory differences cause them to struggle to do what they want and to live a meaningful life. She thought: "As Robyn is helping her clients individually, why not find out if her clinic could help my team get from great to even more amazing: Regulated, actively choosing their sensation, accessing all their knowledge and expertise, and not burned out!"

Grasping what she was seeking hit me with the energy and excitement of fireworks. "Yes! Let's do this!" Let's support a group of helping professionals who want to help more, by showing them that, deep in their souls, they are enough, so they won't be worn out all the time. I could just see it: ripples of hope, change, and love moving through a small company and then spreading beyond.

Our world needs help, the kind of help that comes from a smile and a hug from a stranger, a group of young people thinking differently and choosing action over despair, an expert choosing curiosity and wonder over judgment, no matter how common the situation. This new way of thinking requires us to reconnect with our internal sensory experiences, partner with our bodies, and adjust our external sensory world when we can to support rejuvenation and regulation. It is more than self-care. Sensory health moves us through survival and into thriving.

So welcome to the journey of sensory wellness! Traveling together on the path to deepen our daily experiences is so wonderful. This book is designed to help you bridge the gap between knowledge and embodied living, paying attention to your body's signals and using them to guide everyday choices, so mind and body work together. *Embodiment* in this context is a process and a path. Karden Rabin, co-founder of the Trauma Research Foundation, defines embodiment as "the act of expanding one's self-awareness to include the felt experience of the body, such as sensory, sensational, emotional and physical experiences, and incorporating that information into one's overall conception and conduct of themselves, their identity, beliefs, behaviors, and ways of being" (2022). In this book, we will explore how bringing sensory information into our thoughts improves our self-awareness, self-regulation, and overall health. Sensory wellness sheds light on our identity, helping us to know more about who we are. Think of *Sensory Wellness* as a guide to blooming into your best self, just like a flower nourished by the right soil, water, and sunlight.

In our fast-paced world, we often find ourselves feeling "exhausterwhelmulated" (exhausted, overwhelmed, and overstimulated all at once), reacting thoughtlessly rather than responding intentionally. Sensory wellness is about leveraging how we process sensation from within our bodies and the world around us to thrive at home and work and in our relationships with ourselves and others. This book will help you move from "I know I should" to "I can, and I want to," empowering you to change the sensations of your daily life.

Each chapter provides a mix of neuroscience, personal reflection, and helpful invitations to deepen your understanding of sensory wellness. I encourage you to make time to fully engage in the integration activities throughout the book and then write your observations and thoughts in the *Sensory Wellness Reflection Journal* (or a blank journal of your own). Look out for both the "Do" and "Reflect" invitations. The body-based learning activities, marked with the label "Do," will support deepening your connection with your body. The thought-provoking questions, marked with the label "Reflect," will connect sensory experiences with your past and create sensory wellness for your future. Honor and listen to your body throughout these activities. It is okay to pause. Your journey thus far will impact the right timing and amount of tuning into your body sensations and reflections. Whether you are a professional, a caregiver, someone seeking personal growth, or any combination of these, this book will equip you with the tools to enhance your regulation, resilience, and overall well-being.

In a world where it is common to be disconnected from those around you and even your own self, we are going counterculture, creating a sensory revolution of connection to ourselves and the world around us—to real reality instead of virtual reality. In my job as an occupational therapist specializing in sensory processing and integration, I have seen the power of sensation in bringing people together, healing deep wounds from the past, and releasing inner joy. And this transformation has not only been for the neurodivergent children who come to the clinic. As I have mentored therapists on the brink of burnout and walked with parents who are at their wits' end, I have seen people tune into themselves so they could not just keep going but also flourish!

I'm on this journey too. I didn't realize what calm felt like, truly, until my late thirties. I had turned off my body signals about hunger and needing to go to the bathroom more often than I had tuned in. And the noisy, demanding world was so loud that I was exhausted from trying to pay attention to my work and my kids. And then it occurred to me: sensory wellness is for everyone and anyone. We can all live a more connected, joy-filled life by leaning into sensation.

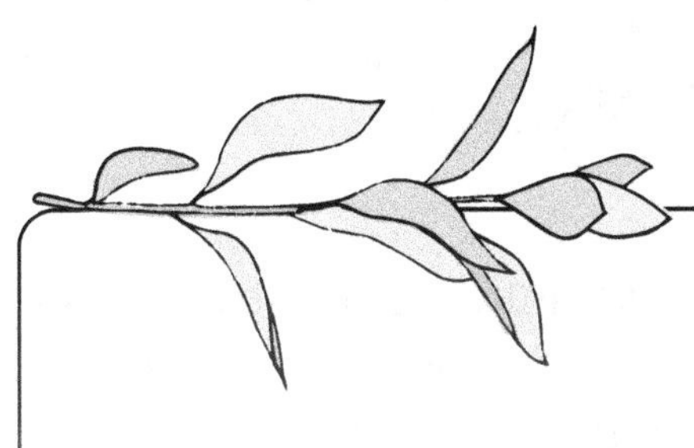

CHAPTER 1

Foundations of Sensory Wellness: Regulation and Self-Awareness

"Until you make the unconscious conscious, it will direct your life and you will call it fate."

~ C. G. Jung ~

Regulation is at the heart of sensory wellness. *Regulation* means noticing your body state (energy, emotions, breathing, stress, awakeness, alertness, etc.) and adjusting—up or down—as you choose to so you can meet the moment. Regulation is not being calm all the time. Calm all the time is not the goal, and it is not even healthy.

A regulated person shifts in and out of calm with fluidity. Our regulation patterns are impacted by the neurology and physiology we were born with and our lifetime of experiences, shaping our interactions with the world. Your current brain-and-body experience of sensation has been shaped by amazing experiences, the happiest moments you can remember, heart-wrenching trauma, and everything in between. When you are regulated and thriving, you are a beautiful flower blooming in all your brilliance, dancing in the breeze. So, let's explore the elements of you thriving and blooming!

Regulation occurs when sense information from your body and the environment travels through your nervous system and into your brain. Your brain directs information in unconscious and conscious ways, predicting and even shifting how you will take in more sensory information. Furthermore, it is not just sensory input in, but a two-way street of our brains and bodies partially determining what sensation we will experience, and of sense information partially determining what happens in our brains and bodies. And all this occurs so fast! Sometimes a gap exists between what happens and what we do. We take a pause, gather our thoughts, and *respond.* Sometimes, what we do is more of a knee-jerk reaction and we think, "I really should have waited to say anything." When we are regulated, we are more likely to respond instead of reacting.

Regulation is actively choosing to utilize the ability to think about a situation a little bit more. You gain wisdom in understanding and managing your behavior, emotions, and/or thoughts in order to pursue your goals: short-term, long-term, or just forming. Regulation includes the ability to act in a way that is consistent with your deepest-held values. Regulation facilitates intentional action.

One of my earliest memories of feeling regulated was a hot summer day when I was around six years old. The mid-morning sun shone down as my dad and I went swimming. It wasn't a splash-all-over, cannonball competition or energetic swim. We floated on our backs and kicked our feet gently as our movement path created the outline of a butterfly shape on the top of the water. My dad glided in one direction, his path outlining the butterfly wing on one side of the butterfly, and I outlined the other wing, moving symmetrically in opposite directions. Connected and separate. Moving and still. Warm and cool. Regulated.

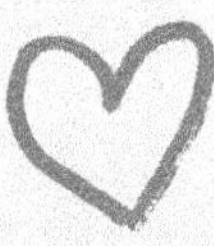

Awareness of your own regulation:

Do: Take a deep breath.

Reflect: When do you remember feeling regulated?

Regulation Under the Surface: Your Autonomic Nervous System

Autonomic Nervous System: A network of nerves throughout your body that manage automatic and mostly unconscious responses in the body to support internal balance, controlling vital functions such as heart rate, blood pressure, breathing, digestion, and sexual arousal. Main divisions are the sympathetic, parasympathetic, and enteric nervous systems.

Sympathetic Nervous System: The part of the autonomic nervous system responsible for the body's response to potentially dangerous situations. It prepares the body to react quickly to stressful or emergency situations, generating a fight, flight, flock, or freeze physiological response including making your heart beat faster, opening your airways, and helping your muscles work. Commonly referred to as the fight-or-flight state or stress response.

Parasympathetic Nervous System: The part of the autonomic nervous system that promotes rest and digestion, helping the body relax and conserve energy after periods of stress or activity, slowing down your heart rate and decreasing your blood pressure. Commonly referred to as the rest-and-digest state or calm response.

Enteric Nervous System: The part of the autonomic nervous system that is made up of a complex network of nerves throughout your digestive system, managing the digestion of food without thinking about the process.

The *autonomic nervous system* plays a crucial role in regulation. It is the body's automatic control system, managing heart rate, breathing, blood pressure, and digestion as you move through the day. Its two main branches—the sympathetic and the parasympathetic—work together: the *sympathetic* (stress response) switches the body into high-alert survival mode when your senses perceive danger, and the *parasympathetic* (calm response) supports the rest and digest state when your senses perceive safety.

The Stress Response

Oprah Winfrey and psychologist Bruce Perry discuss increased sympathetic activation being one of four responses: fight, flight (move away), flock (go to friends), or freeze, in the book *What Happened to You?* (2021).

Of these four responses, one of the least familiar is *freeze.* Freeze is like an opossum playing dead. It's an actual physiological freeze, where your heart rate goes way down, because your body is literally trying to play dead. Pretty intense.

We can observe the stress response inside the body from outside clues. When I was growing up, my parents were avid runners, and I have many fond memories of cheering them on in races and exploring new trails with them. One fall day when I was about 13, my dad got back from a run near our house, and something was wrong. I could tell immediately from the way his body moved as he walked towards the front door. My mom and I ran towards the door and saw his neck

Autonomic Nervous System

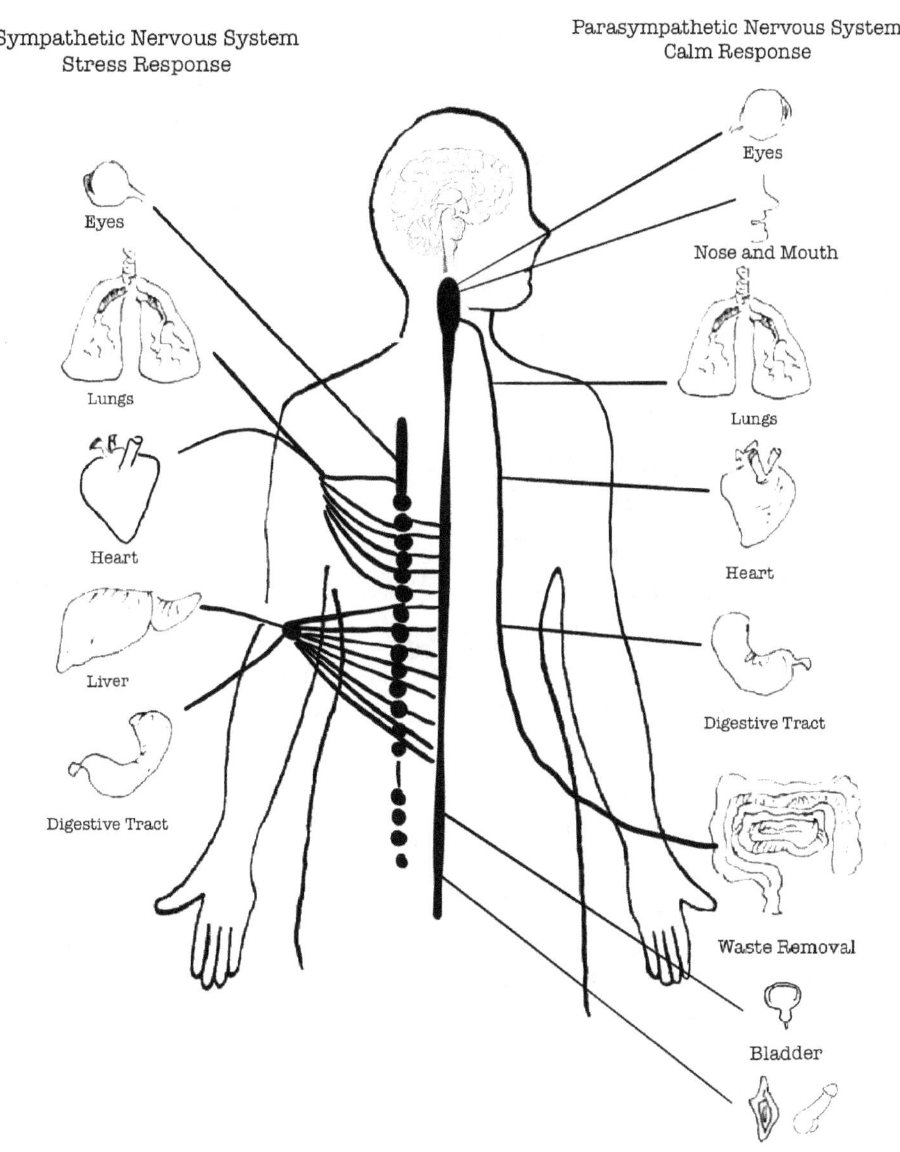

swelling up quickly. Dad had been stung by bees while he was running, and this was his biggest allergic reaction ever! As my mom led my dad to the car, I gathered my sisters and grabbed the allergy medicine out of the cabinet. We got to the emergency room quickly, and my dad was rushed into the resuscitation bay. He was having a hard time breathing, and his ear was puffed up like nothing I had ever seen. My job, as the big sister, was to keep an eye on my sisters in the waiting room while they were watching a Disney movie playing on the television (I still don't love *Rescuers Down Under* because it was playing that day). When my mom came out to the waiting room to check in, I picked up the signs of the stress response even though I didn't know what they were officially. As I recall the memory, I can see the pupils of her eyes dilated, bigger than ever. I slipped my hand in hers and felt the wetness of sweat from the stress. Her body perceived the danger and reacted accordingly. And while the stress response decreased in all of us as my dad began to breathe again, this memory has stayed (and my dad got an epi-pen).

When an autistic child I worked with in our clinic would come in for therapy sessions, his pupils would be so big I could barely see the color of his irises. The intensity of the sensations from the car ride to the clinic mixed with the sensations from his own body drove his stress response through the roof! As we played a make-believe version of garbage truck driver with swings, bean bags, scooter boards, and weighted balls, I could start to see the brown color of his eyes. The shrinking of his pupils and the blooming of his irises was a real, observable physical response showing the regulation process had kicked in with the shift of the autonomic nervous system balance.

Other things that happen to your body in a stress response:

- ✦ Heart rate increases to pump blood to your muscles faster.
- ✦ Palms become sweaty to help cool the body.
- ✦ Lung muscles relax to let in as much oxygen as possible.
- ✦ Blood goes straight out to your muscles, so you can run faster and get away from danger.
- ✦ Immune system goes into a higher gear. This may sound like a good thing, but if a person's immune system is being activated often every day, it is being overworked and will become compromised. Then a person will start getting sick all the time. This can be a problem long term.

Quick sympathetic activation in a moment of danger is essential, but it can be unhelpful when the response is really big and the danger is gone or wasn't ever there. So we need to learn to regulate. However, that can be harder than it sounds, as we can see when we look into the brain activity of someone with a triggered stress response. In many situations, the higher-level thinking networks in the brain (areas of the brain that often communicate with each other and work together to help us plan and achieve goals in life) are not working well or at all when the fight, flight, flock, or freeze response occurs, wiping out logical thinking support from your brain. So reasoning and weighing out decisions and their implications for the future are pretty offline. And if you are not aware that your stress response is activated, you will also likely not be aware if someone else is in an activated state too. This mix of two people trying to interact, problem solve, and get through a day while in an activated sympathetic response can damage their relationship, leading to lots of pain and misunderstanding. So side note, if you hear someone saying extreme words like "always" and "never," they are likely having an increased stress response (like parents at odds about how to treat their picky eater), and waiting to solve problems or resolve a conflict may be a good idea.

Why may your body's stress response increase if no bear is chasing you?

- Someone yells at you.
- A car accident happens right in front of you.
- You see something you are scared of.
- Something happens in your environment or in your body that reminds you of a past trauma.
- Your body and brain have big responses to sounds, and someone unexpectedly turns on the vacuum cleaner.

Nerves: Cells in your body that carry messages (electrical signals) between your brain and the rest of your body. Nerves are involved in everything you do, think, and feel.

Neurotransmitters: Chemicals produced by nerve cells when nerves are activated (fire) helping nerves talk to other nerves, muscles, and glands. Neurotransmitters communicate between cells, transfer information, and impact body functions, including mood, appetite, sleep, memory, motor coordination. Examples include dopamine, serotonin, norepinephrine, glutamate, and GABA.

The stress response causes a huge release of the neurotransmitter norepinephrine. According to the Cleveland Clinic, low levels of norepinephrine can lead to anxiety, depression, attention challenges, headaches, memory problems, and sleep disturbances. High levels of norepinephrine can result in high blood pressure, rapid heartbeat, excessive sweating, cold skin, severe headaches, and nervousness. So, we don't want to create a lifestyle where there is no sympathetic activation, and we also do not want to constantly be in a state of sympathetic overdrive: fight, flight, flock, or freeze. Just as plants need the sun to shine but would not do well if the sun were to shine day and night, we need balance. On this journey of sensory wellness, self-awareness is one of the first sprouts of growth.

Awareness of your own stress response:

Do: Feel the palms of your hands. How much moisture do you notice?

Reflect: When have you experienced a stress response?

The Calm Response

Now for the other component of the autonomic nervous system, the *parasympathetic* or calm response. Remember playground teeter-totters? As one side goes up, the other side goes down. That is a good illustration for the autonomic nervous system. Parasympathetic activation (the calm response) is on one side of the teeter-totter, and sympathetic activation (the stress response) is on the other, with a continuum of activation. As one goes up, the other goes down, and they can be pretty balanced, with one side being only slightly higher than the other. If the stress response is slightly activated, for example, I may feel the sweat on my upper lip (a sign of sympathetic activation) but not have a full-blown panic attack (because my parasympathetic system is not all the way inactive), meaning my teeter-totter is only slightly off balance. The teeter-totter illustration helps explain the interaction between the two responses in a simplified form, as the two systems are not always perfectly inversely activated, but this is a good start to understanding the relationship between the stress and calm responses.

Signs of parasympathetic activation include a decreased breathing rate, a decreased heart rate, and increased digestion. This makes sense because if you have a bear chasing you and you're trying to get away as fast as possible, whether or not you absorb the protein from the hot dog you ate that day doesn't really matter in regard to keeping you alive. Your body shuts down digestion to focus on running fast and getting away. However, if you are experiencing stress responses intensely and often, your body is always trying to get away from scary bears and cannot be bothered with absorbing the nutrients from the food you're eating even if you are eating the most amazingly nutritious meals. This is part of the reason some of the neurodivergent people I get to work with as an occupational therapist are constipated often, especially when they are in a new place: Life is stressful! Constipation is a sign of decreased digestion. You need increased parasympathetic activation to fully absorb nutrients into your body. Luckily, we can strategically use some types of sensation in order to increase the calm response. (Also, orgasms occur when you have increased parasympathetic activation. So if you are in a stress response state all the time, you are less likely to have an orgasm during intimacy. That's no fun!)

Remember, your stress and calm responses are turned up and down without you even thinking about it. That means that unless you actively try to notice these components or

Detection of your own calm response:

Do: Breathe in and then breathe out longer than you breathed in.

Reflect: When did you experience an increased calm response?

your response gets so big that it forces you to pay attention to it, you may be unaware of what is happening in your autonomic nervous system, even though your stress response is impacting the way you interact with the world around you and the sensations within you. So, what may happen to get your attention?

- ✦ You lose your temper with a loved one.
- ✦ Your health starts breaking down.
- ✦ Your world starts falling apart.
- ✦ You have a panic attack.
- ✦ You have a heart attack.
- ✦ Your addiction gets so bad that you lose your job or your family or both.

But until something big happens, many people go through their daily lives not noticing the fluctuations of their autonomic nervous system. Only after they experience one of these major life events, might they start paying attention to their stress responses. When we repeatedly ignore our body signals, we, as a society and across many cultures, are often not thriving. We can start listening to our own stress responses sooner and make adjustments in our lives.

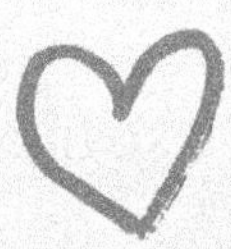

Increasing awareness of your stress response:

Do: Ask a safe person to touch your arm or hand with a light touch, drawing a curved line in an S shape. Then, ask them to give you a hug or a shoulder rub. What did you notice in your body during each of these sensory experiences?

Reflect: What is a common first clue in your body that your stress response is turning up?

How can we tell if our bodies are doing a good job shifting between increasing stress and calm responses? The goal is *not* that the stress and calm responses are balanced. Just like a car does not drive and stop well if both the gas and brake peddles are pushed down at the same time, we don't want both the stress and calm response activated. Health does include good stress, in the right measure and at the right time. We want the right response (stress or calm) to lead at the right time. Scientists have studied the connection between heart rate variability, the fluctuation in time between heartbeats, and overall health. Heart rate variability is a marker of resilience, ability to roll with changes in life, fitness, and maintaining health when life is stressful. If your nervous system is moving between increased stress and calm responses like the ebb and flow of ocean waves, your heart rate will vary. Our brains and bodies are happiest when our heart rate goes up and down regularly, but not excessively, and comes back to our baseline throughout the day and night. And heart rate variability is easily trackable! You can track your own heart rate variability as you read through *Sensory Wellness* and complete the integration activities.

Here's a concrete example of heart rate variability in real time for multiple people in the same situation. My family and I got to go swim with manta rays, and it was an amazing experience! One manta ray swam toward me, beautifully dancing in the water, and then he swam up toward the surface so close to me that our bellies almost touched! Then he swam away. I love the ocean and marine animals, and, in that moment, I could feel my heart beating really fast. Then I looked over at my daughter, Bethany, who was around eight years old at the time. She was very scared, to the point of being adamant that she did not want to be there. The wooziness of being on a boat, the deep, dark ocean below, and the safety talk had all pushed her past the excitement of seeing some of her favorite animals and into a big stress response, including a tricky combination of flight and freeze responses. She wanted out of there: to snap her fingers and be off the boat. And her body was immobilized. My heart started beating even faster when I saw the fear in her eyes and her white knuckles. Then I looked over at my son, Isaac, and he was grinning ear to ear, eyes huge, excited in a best-day-ever kind of way. At that point my heart rate went down as I reflected on being his mom and facilitating this experience for him. That was how the whole manta ray experience went: a couple of hours of emotions coming and going, heart rate going up and down. Your ability to adapt and respond to change indicates health, not your ability to stop or control change. Side note: my daughter ended up being happy she went and also sure she wouldn't go again.

"The only constant in life is change."

- Heraclitus -

We can improve our heart rate variability and our overall wellness in a variety of ways rooted in sensation, integration, and regulation. Improved regulation not only improves your heart rate variability, it affects your brain connections and function, too! Regulation is working toward lining up what you're doing daily with where you want to go long term.

Tuning into heart rate variability:

Do: Notice your heartbeat. Where can you detect it in your body?
Reflect: Check if your phone has any heart rate variability data on it. See if the data shown matches with some of your memories of the last week or so. If your phone does not have heart rate variability data on it, you can look into some low-cost heart rate variability tracking options. Lots of options available!

Self-Awareness

Self-awareness is pivotal in supporting our emotional flow, regulation and connection with others. A person *can* go from really upset to not upset without being aware of themself. But this process is longer and harder. Much harder. *Self-awareness* is your ability to interpret and make sense of your physical sensations, thoughts, emotions, actions and behaviors, desires, and intentions. Self-awareness is your overall perception of yourself and also how you impact others. What's going on in your head when you look in the mirror is a part of self-awareness. Counter-intuitively, self-awareness is not a "more is always better" capacity. Research shows that people who are too self-aware without regulation capability are at a higher risk for anxiety and depression. Throughout *Sensory Wellness*, we will strategically build self-awareness while also increasing our regulation know-how in order to support healthy growth.

Developing more self-awareness

Do: Bring your attention to your body, one area at a time. Start with your head and work your way down, noticing any tightness, pain, warmth, tension, etc.

Reflect: Make a list of all the emotions you have felt in the last couple of days.

SECTION 2

Sensory Systems in Daily Life

"My advice is: You always have to keep persevering."

- Temple Grandin -

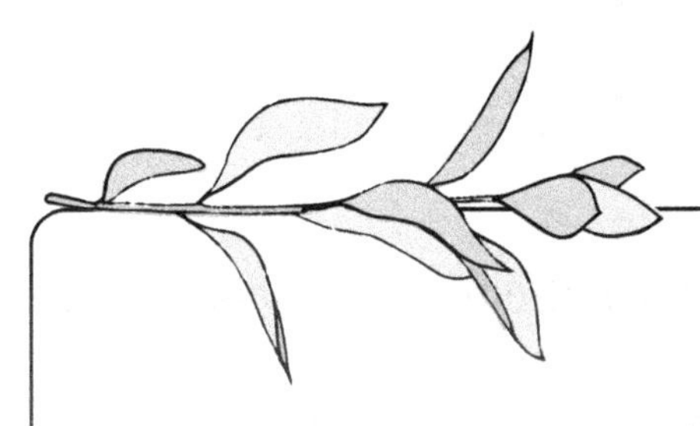

CHAPTER 2

Sensory Overview

"The senses, being the explorers of the world, open the way to knowledge."

- Maria Montessori -

Sensory wellness is all about sensations coming from within and from outside your body impacting your actions. Interestingly, two people can have the same sensory experience and interpret it completely differently. For some people, a sensory experience can be super fun, like my son having the time of his life on a roller coaster. For others, though, it can be absolutely terrifying, like my daughter even thinking about going on the roller coaster or having to watch people go on the roller coaster. Understanding that the same sensation can feel very different to two people requires self-awareness and perspective taking. Emotional maturity helps us understand and realize that while we may be having a lot of fun at a party, someone else may not be enjoying the party at all. More knowledge of sensory processing and integration can help expand, integrate, and apply these concepts to everyday life, helping us take care of ourselves and connect with others!

The power of sensation really hit home for me at the birthday party for my son's friend when the boys were about five years old. The party had a *Cars* theme, as it was shortly after the movie came out, and the cupcakes were decorated with the little *Cars* figurines. As all the birthday boy's little friends finished singing the "Happy Birthday" song with their silly "and many more" additions, the birthday boy looked up at his mother with big tears starting to spill out of his eyes. I heard him say, "Momma, I totally want to eat the cupcake, but there's all the frosting in the way. It's so sticky and gross. And I just...I don't know what to do."

He was so sweet, and I could feel his mother's heart hurting for her son, bewildered by his actions. She gave him a hug and quickly swiped off the offending frosting. The boy ate his plain cupcake and went back to enjoying his birthday party. The mom shared with me later that it was at that moment that she realized something was different; he wasn't just a picky eater. He wanted to eat the cupcake, but he couldn't. She resolved to make sure he received the help he needed.

***Sensory Modulation*:** The brain perceiving, regulating, and responding to sensation in order help a person participate in meaningful daily life activities. Sensory modulation includes filtering out some sensations while attending to others.

We all take in sensory information differently, and sensation creates experience. Sensory information comes in through 20+ senses (depending on how you count various types of receptors and define systems), is registered by our brain, and then is modulated. *Modulation* means our body and brain decide if the sensation is taking up too much or too little of our brain's operating power. Can I focus and interact with others with this amount of sensation? Sometimes without even consciously thinking about it, we adjust the amount and intensity of incoming information. I often get in the car in the morning and turn down the volume on my music without thinking about it because morning me does not prefer the volume nighttime me loves. Sometimes familiar sensation levels shift without us consciously paying attention to them: like the air conditioner turning on and off and blowing the fabric of our clothes toward and away from our skin.

And other times the slightest change in sensation can send us into full fight, flight, flock, or freeze mode: like the change in rhythm of my niece's voice when she went from happily playing on the playground to almost falling from a high platform. I had been sitting on a bench talking to another parent, heard my niece's abruptly changed voice, and without even thinking dashed to be right below to catch her if she should fall.

Our brain and body constantly team up to adjust many different kinds of sensation and interpret all the sensory information and details uniquely, making each of us deeply individual. Let's explore some of the major sensory systems and bring conscious awareness to our own sensory processing.

Exteroception and Interoception

Remember those cute little songs about the five senses we learned in kindergarten? Sight, Sound, Smell, Taste, and Touch? Those are just the beginning of the story. Many different specialized cell types take in sensory information, which are grouped to create sensory systems. Inside-the-body signals are interoceptive senses and outside-the-body signals are exteroceptive. Different parts of the brain and networks handle each.

Exteroception: Sensation that represents perception of information outside your body.

Interoception: Sensation that represents perception of information inside your body.

We are constantly gathering and feeling both types of signals all the time. Past experiences affect how you notice and read sensation, which also shapes your connections with others. If something wonderful happened the last time I ate watermelon, my brain will likely interpret the taste of watermelon as amazing the next time I eat it *and* be on the lookout for another good thing happening! The brain is a powerful prediction machine, looking for sensory information to confirm or change our guess about what is going to happen. My brain gets the message from my eyes: I just saw a shade of pink that matches with the last delicious watermelon I ate! My temperature receptors tell my brain this watermelon I am holding is chilled to my blissful delight. Almost instantaneously, my brain predicts: this is going to be a wonderful experience! The brain's predictions constantly adjust with new experiences: adapting and creating meaning to help us navigate daily life.

The good news: you can change how you interpret sensations, and you can change sensation within your body and your environment. You may not control the whole world, but you can reshape your sensory world—and your daily experience.

Experiencing and envisioning your sensational life:

Do: Take five minutes (or more) and do something you sensationally love! Anything: use your favorite scented lotion, go for a walk, take a nap, soak in a bath, listen to a song. Stay present and deeply feel. If your thoughts wander or you feel the urge to pick up your phone and check something, gently and kindly bring yourself back.

Reflect: Envision your ideal sensory day. You wake up and what do you want to hear? What would you like to smell? What is the temperature of the air? What do you want to see on the walls? What do you want to see out the window? What is your bathroom like? What is in your closet? You look at yourself in the mirror and you can look however you want. How would you like to look today? You go down to breakfast. Who is at the table? What do you eat? Then, where do you go? How does the day wrap up? Record your vision in the *Sensory Wellness Reflection Journal* or download and write your vision on the Ideal Sensory Day resource, free on my website.

But before we focus on reshaping your sensory world, in the next several chapters we will dive into some of the sensory systems and get to know them more. While the information on the sensory systems is evidence-based and interesting from a science perspective, let's not just spend precious time thinking about these sensory systems as a purely cerebral lesson. Let's ground ourselves in sensation to change lives: our own first, and then the lives of those around us.

As we learn about each sensory system, take a moment to reflect on familiar sensations and write down one of your favorite sensations in the *Sensory Wellness Reflection Journal* or your notebook. For instance, for the visual system, one of my favorite visual sensations is seeing dolphins jumping through water as I look out at the open ocean past the nose of my surfboard. This image makes my heart sing! Of all the visual images I love, this scene is the first one that jumps into my mind.

Sensation Flower

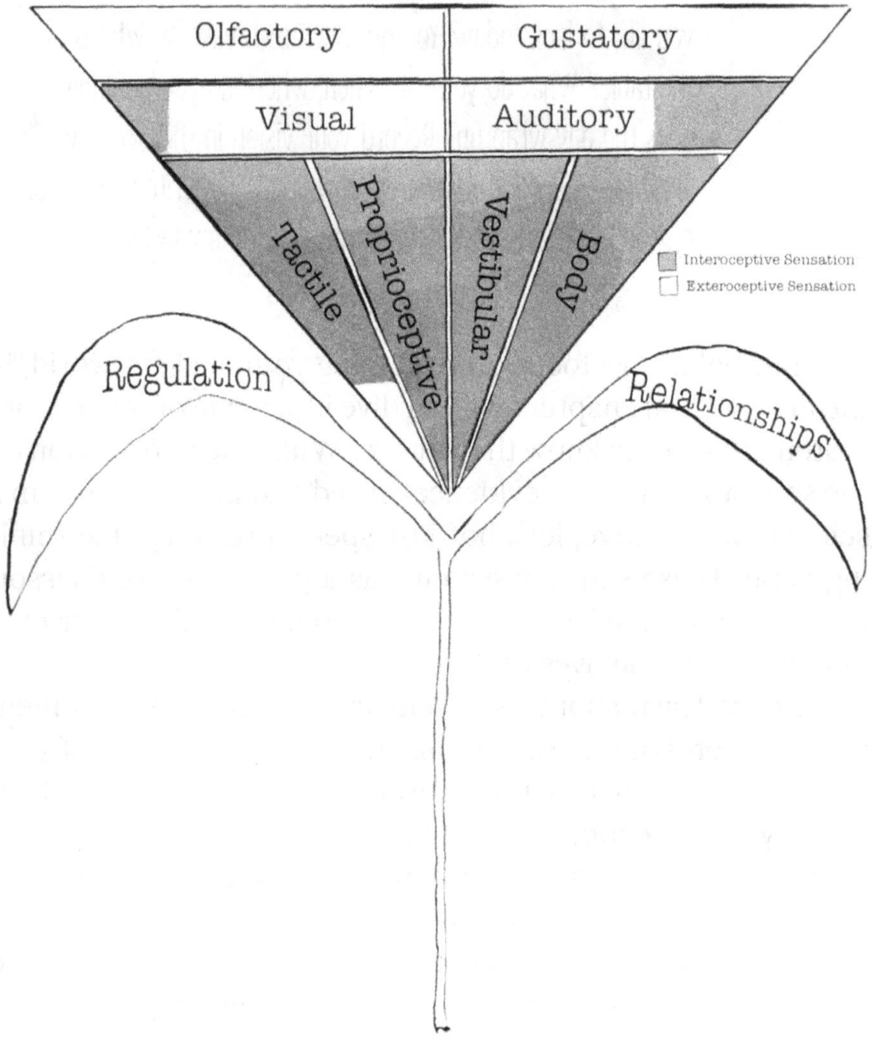

Don't overthink it, and don't skip the reflection invitations. Take a moment for each sensory system and fully imagine the sensation you enjoy. Noting a favorite sensation is a crucial part of the journey of sensory wellness.

The other application activity I will guide you in as we go through the sensory systems is reflecting on your ideal amount of sensation for that specific system. If you could wave a magic wand and all the people in your life would agree with you and support that level of sensation, what kind and how much of that type of sensation would you prefer? For instance, if you could cook whatever you want for dinner and everyone in your home would be okay with your choice, would you make a flavorful meal or a more bland one? Pasta or protein? You will rate your preference for each sensory system on a scale of **1** to **10**, with **10** being the most of that kind of sensation you could ever imagine, and **1** being almost none, just barely even existing in your world. Intensity, predictability, order, and variability can all contribute to your rating. The resource "My Sensory World" will help guide you through this activity and provides a place to record your thoughts. You can use these pages in your *Sensory Wellness Reflection Journal* or find "My Sensory World" in the resources section of my website.

Then, the last step we'll do for each of the eight sensory systems we're going to talk about is marking down how much of that type of sensation is in your current reality. When you think about the places you normally do life, how much of that kind of input is around you? We will use the same scale of 1 to 10. Again, go with your gut response. Don't worry about being exact. Let's not bring out a sound meter to measure exactly how many decibels of sound are in your world hour by hour. On our **1** to **10** scale, if you have more order and less unpredictability within that type of sensation, you might be on the lower side of the continuum and closer to a **1**. If you currently experience a bit more unpredictable sensation with more intensity, you may be rating yourself closer to a **10**.

Why am I suggesting you do these activities as part of this book? These application activities are foundational work to help you thrive *and* will make the sensory tools section of this book easier. When you use sensation to adjust your energy level to match what you need or want to do, you can move through your life more regulated and healthier. You will start to analyze: what can I incorporate into my environment and my routine that will support the difference between the sensation in my current world and my preferred sensory levels? We are not going to always have our perfect day, but we can absolutely make the day a bit better by taking a moment to chew a piece of gum, not because of bad breath or to pop our ears during a drive or flight to combat the effects of an elevation change, but because it will increase a proprioceptive sensation that increases the release of feel-good chemicals in our brains. *Knowing more can improve our sensory wellness and thus our lives.*

Sensory Receptors: Specialized cells and nerve endings that detect sense information about the internal and external environment.

Also, to help you grow into a place where you are powerfully adjusting sensation, I want to tell you a little bit about where the receptors are for the different sensory systems. Some are super obvious, like visual receptors in the eye. But some of the sensory receptors are not as commonly known. For instance, the vestibular (balance and movement) receptors are in your inner ear. When you move your head, you activate your balance and movement system. So, if your head position isn't changing, it doesn't matter if your foot is moving.

You are not increasing vestibular input. No vestibular receptors exist in your foot. We will go through the details about the sensory receptors so you can create your own sensory supportive lifestyle.

One more thing! You are not just receiving sensation from your world and reacting to it; you are actually shifting how you are perceiving the sensation around you based on your neurophysiology and your past experiences. So, for instance, when I hold a cup of hot tea made just as my grandmother made it when I was growing up, I perceive the sensory data of our interactions together with a warmer, more friendly touch than if I were drinking something cold. We can influence the sensory information we detect in the environment around us and how we will determine the meaning of that input. Powerful.

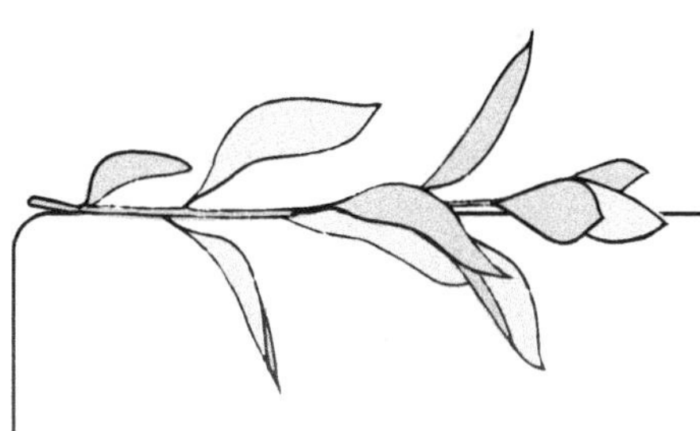

CHAPTER 3

The Visual/Sight System

"We do not see things as they are, we see them as we are."

- Anaïs Nin -

The sense of sight takes a long time to develop after you are born. Beginning around day 33 in your mother's womb, your little sensory receptors for vision (photoreceptors) started forming. *Visual acuity* (detailed vision) is developed between age five and 15 years old. Most children can see 20 feet away by the age of five.

Returning to the autonomic nervous system from chapter 1, your entire visual system reconfigures during a stress response in order to focus on long-range and motion detection, rather than on little details, accurate depth perception, and color gradients. You don't need to know the color of the bear, or whether it is male or female, in order to get away from danger as fast as you can.

Our visual system shift makes complete sense in a survival world and can present a difficult challenge in a classroom or everyday life. A kindergartener may not feel safe for lots of reasons. He may not feel safe because of drug exposure in utero impacting his brain development. Or maybe he

Visual System

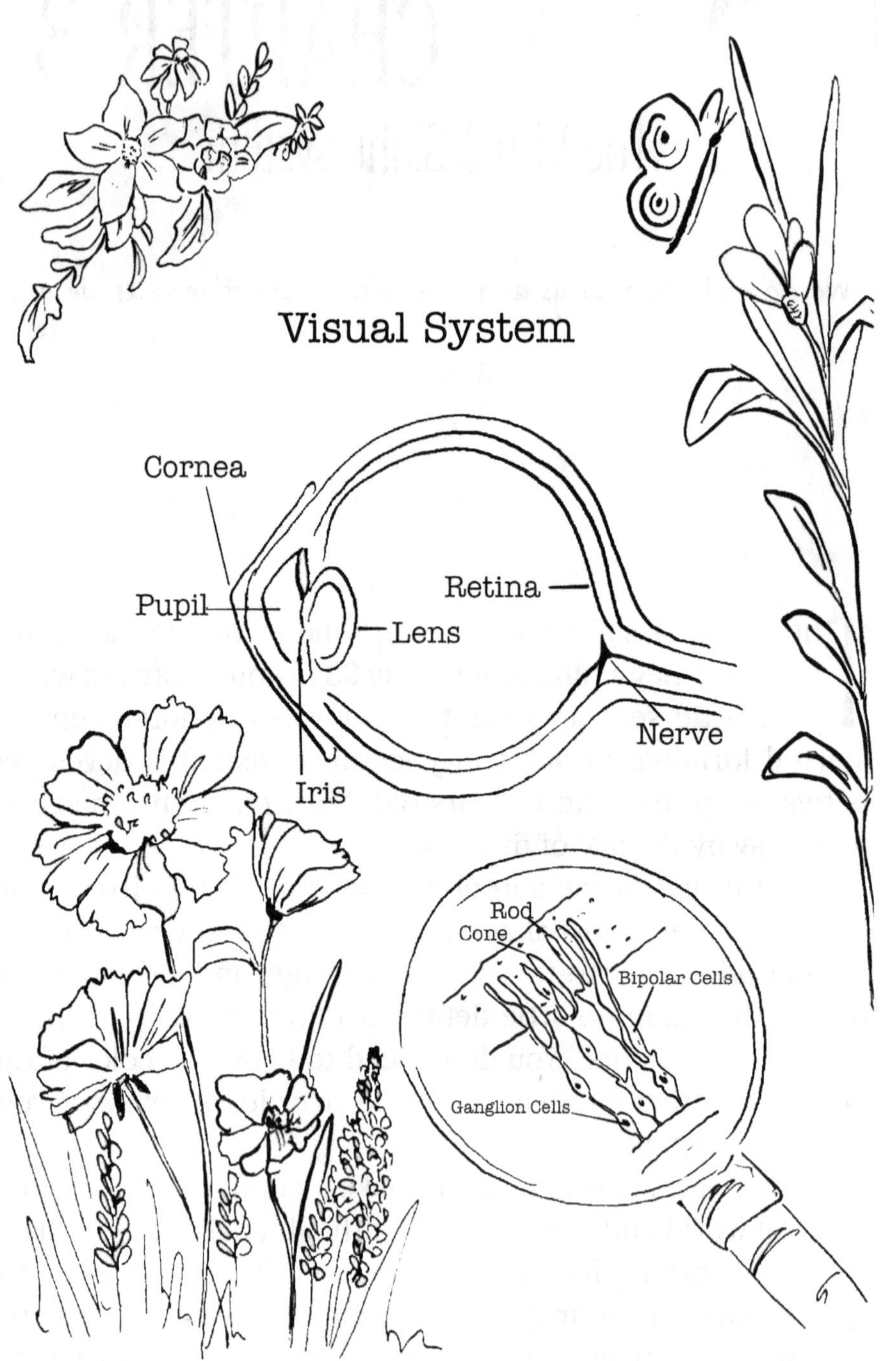

experienced abuse at home on a green couch, and the green classroom walls remind his nervous system of horrific events. Or maybe he is autistic and the student artwork on the walls paired with the social interaction expectations of the school day are too much. When a child does not feel safe, the brain shifts into threat mode, and the stress response increases. The eyes still work, but the child's attention and near-focus do not lock onto fine details—letters on a page, small symbols, or subtle visual cues, such as a reassuring glance from a teacher or a friendly wave from a classmate. Stress can widen the pupils, make focusing jumpy, and narrow attention toward possible danger, hindering the child's ability to pay attention to learning tasks. So even with excellent teaching and engaging activities, a frightened child will miss important visual details because the stress response is driving how the brain works.

If you have been in a constant state of survival mode, you may see changes in what you want in your visual world as you begin to move toward sensory wellness, enjoying more of the beauty of the world around you. When I'm paddling on water after surfing a beautiful wave and I see the reflections of the sunrise and the patterns of the colors of the light dancing with the fluctuations of the currents and the breeze, I greatly appreciate the visual receptors in my eyes.

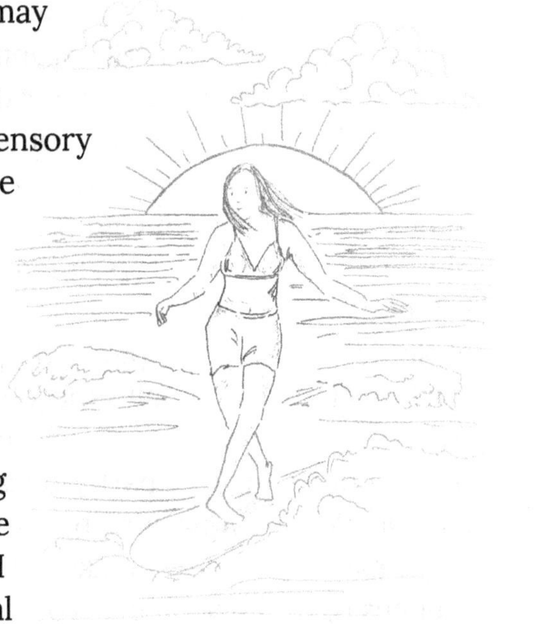

Tuning into your visual system:

Do: Take a moment to absorb and become conscious of all the visual information around you. Notice what happens to your breathing when you pause doing life and focus on your visual sensory world.
Reflect: What visual sensations do you absolutely love?

Rate Your Preferences

Turn to the "My Sensory World" resource on pages 16 and 17 in the *Sensory Wellness Reflection Journal* or download the resource from my website. Think about whether you prefer a lot of visual information or a little visual information. You may be close to a **10** on the rating scale if you have painted the rooms in your house vibrant colors, hung lots of pictures on the walls, and posted many different mementos (pictures, quotes, and cards) on the front of your refrigerator. Think about your preference for your countertops in your house. If your preference is that the counters have absolutely nothing on them, you're maybe closer to a **1** for the amount of visual information you like in your life. If you are not bothered by lots of items on your counters, it may be because your preference is lots of visual information. How much do you care about or notice if pictures are perfectly parallel to the roof line and the floor line and equally spaced? You can absolutely change your answers, and your sensory preferences will likely change throughout your life, partly because your sensory receptors change. Record your current visual sensation preference.

Resist the urge to make guesses about the sensory preferences of other people in your close circle, family members, and loved ones. Many professionals and caregivers spend so much time thinking about those around them that we neglect to take care of ourselves, blocking out and even ignoring sensory clues about what we need in order to keep helping those around us. You can also talk with those in your close circle about their sensory preferences, and I've included places to record their answers in the appendix of the companion journal. Just wait until after you have started thinking about your own sensory preferences before you start asking others about theirs in a loving, kind, and curious way. You may be surprised by their preferences as well as your own! Part of the joy of getting to know yourself and others in a sensational way is understanding that sensory preferences change over time.

Your Current Reality

Now switching gears: what is your current reality of the amount of visual information in your life? Record this on your "My Sensory World" resource as well. Think about your house, your kitchen, your living room, your bedroom, your office area, and your desk. How much visual information is in your everyday environment? Remember: no wrong answers here. Our differences are what make the world a beautiful and wonderful place!

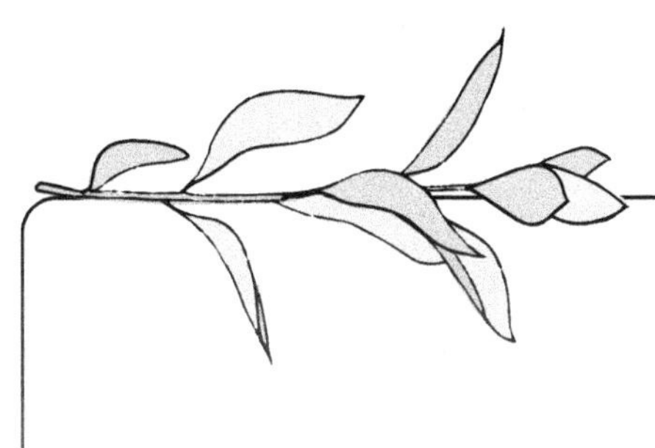

CHAPTER 4

The Auditory/Sound System

"The earth laughs in flowers."

- Ralph Waldo Emerson -

On the hearing side of things, auditory receptors are later than visual receptors to start developing, around week 18. The auditory system is fully developed much sooner than the visual system, at around five to six months old. At 28 weeks in the womb, a baby can tell a difference between their parents' voices and has different brain and body responses to each caregiver. It's absolutely amazing!

The auditory receptors are in your inner ear and are not simply on or off. These receptors send different strengths of messages to the brain depending on the intensity of the auditory information, called graded responses. The hair cell receptors and vibration of little bones in the ear do not just say, "You heard it. Yes, sound," but instead tell your brain the loudness and frequency (high or low notes) of the sound quickly enough that you can use the information to tell where the sound came from as well.

I have a music pillow that helps me to sleep at night, and it vibrates the auditory information only to me. It does not

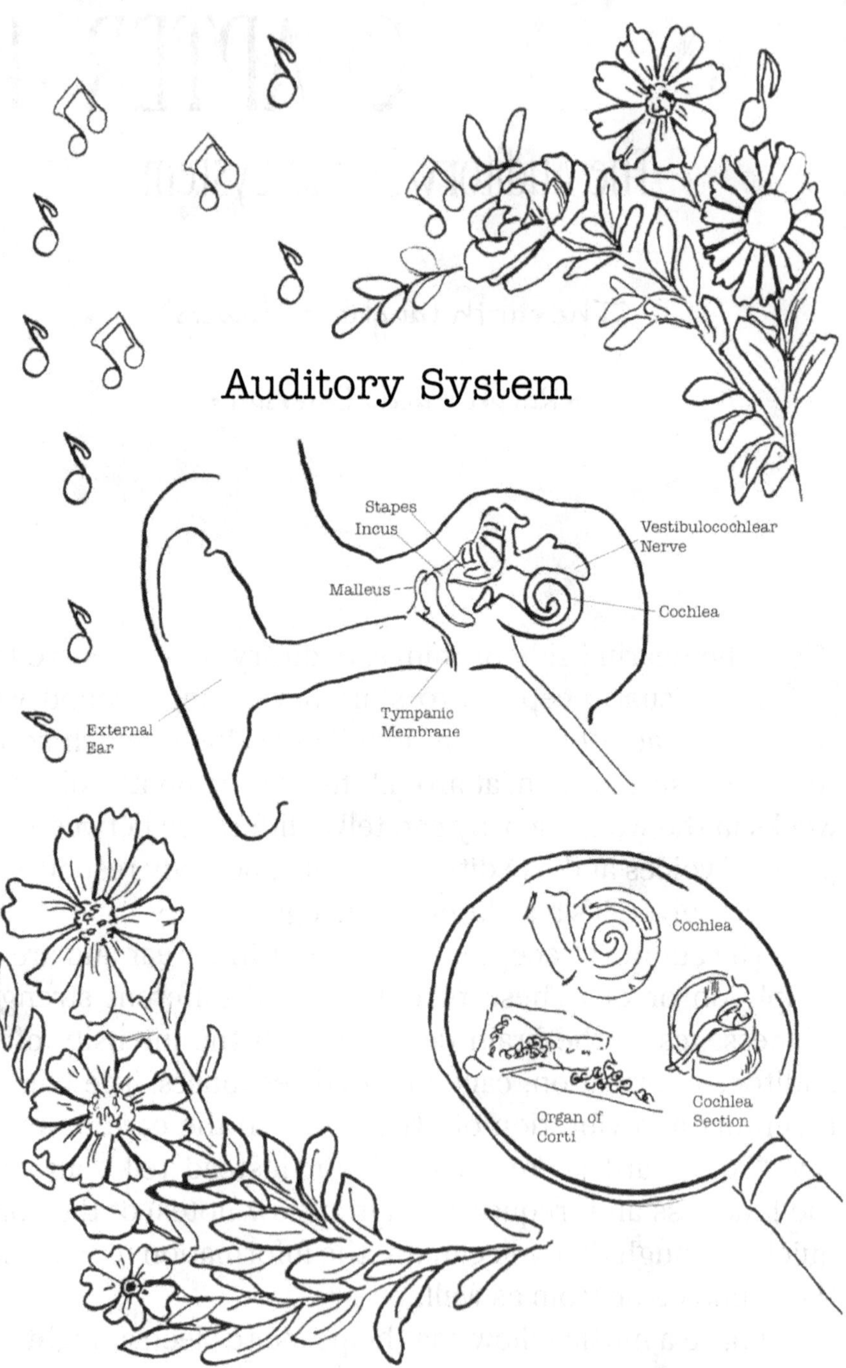

Auditory System
Stapes
Incus
Malleus
Vestibulocochlear Nerve
Cochlea
External Ear
Tympanic Membrane
Cochlea
Organ of Corti
Cochlea Section

have any sound frequencies coming through the air. When my head is on my pillow, I hear and perceive the ocean waves and classical music. When my head is not on it, I don't hear it at all because it's not vibrating my bones. And no one else in the room can hear it unless their head is on my pillow too.

I love the sound of babies and toddlers giggling. Can you hear the magic in their laughter? Awe, wonder, curiosity, and joy! I can't stop the smiling when I hear a baby giggling and playing peek-a-boo with their parent.

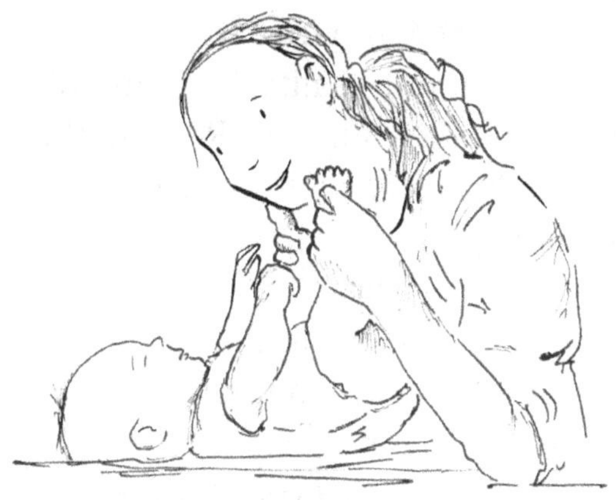

Do: Take a moment to absorb and become conscious of all the auditory information around you.
Reflect: What auditory sensations do you love?

Rate Your Preferences

You may be close to a **10** for auditory preference if you love having televisions and computers playing different shows in lots of rooms of your house at the same time or playing shows or music all day. Preferring a high volume may put you closer to a **10** as well. You may be closer to a **1** if you turn down the volume level or turn everything off when you are really trying to focus on something. Your ideal auditory number may be based less on volume, and more on the speed, beat, and/or pitch. A **10** would be music with various tempo levels or fast tempos, and a **1** would be tempos that are more constant or slower than 60 beats per minute (an average heart rate). Lower musical notes and little change in notes may be part of why your ideal auditory input level is closer to a 1. Note your ideal amount of auditory information.

Your Current Reality

Now explore your current reality in terms of the amount of auditory information in your life. Record this on your "My Sensory World" resource as well. Do you teach in a full classroom of busy elementary students? Do you drive or ride a train through a bustling city? Are you taking care of multiple toddlers who seem to love loud toys and never nap at the same time? Do you work on a computer with noise-cancelling headphones on or operate heavy machinery? Rate the current level of all the sounds in your everyday life.

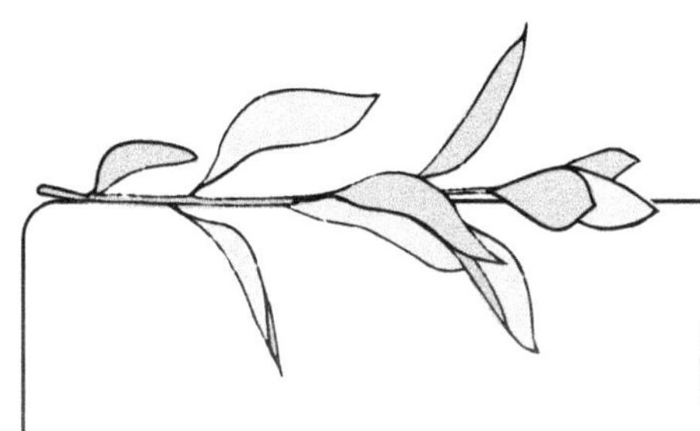

CHAPTER 5

The Tactile/Touch System

"Touch comes before sight, before speech. It is the first language and the last, and it always tells the truth."

- Margaret Atwood -

The tactile or touch system is your first sensory system to develop and start working. Babies start feeling some touch information seven to eight weeks into their time in the womb—early on! Your tactile system is fully functional at 32 weeks into development and has the most different kinds of specialized cell receptors taking in touch information different ways (See Tactile Receptors illustration). The different kinds of *physical change receptors* (*mechanoreceptors*) tell you really important information, such as a spider is crawling on your arm close to your elbow. *Temperature receptors* (*thermoreceptors*) tell you where you are feeling warm or cold. Lastly, *pain receptors* in your skin (*nociceptors*) alert your brain to pain related to temperature, pressure, and chemicals. The *tactile system* is a complex symphony of information signaling your brain. The body devotes a lot of energy to the tactile system because this system is crucial in keeping us safe. On a very basic level, depending on what part of the world you are in, you need to know if a tick (Ew!) is crawling up your arm

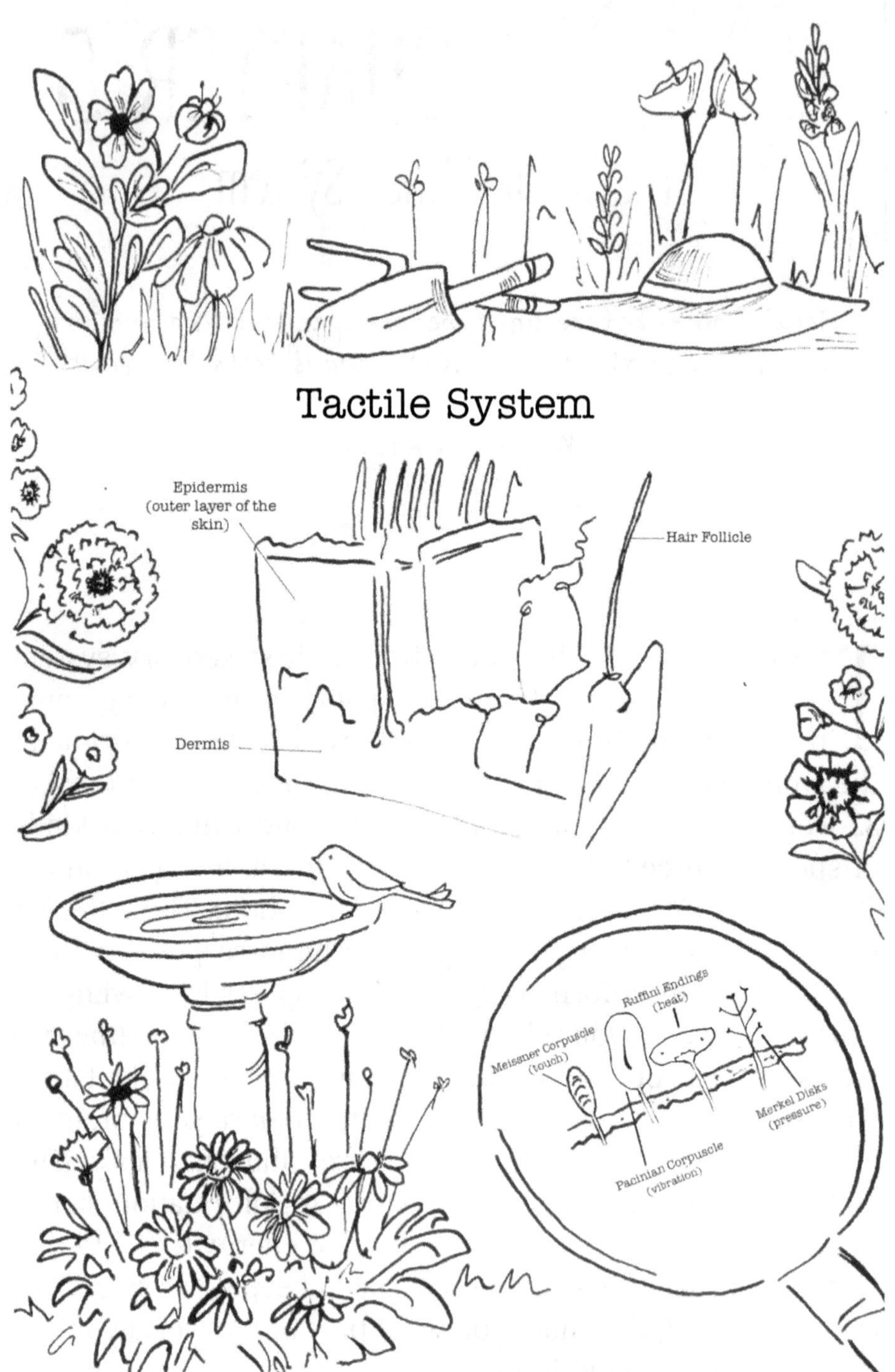
Tactile System
Epidermis
(outer layer of the
skin)
Hair Follicle
Dermis
Ruffini Endings
(heat)
Meissner Corpuscle
(touch)
Merkel Disks
(pressure)
Pacinian Corpuscle
(vibration)

and what type of tick it may be, because it could hurt you very quickly. The tactile system is in the present: right here, right now, keeping us alive.

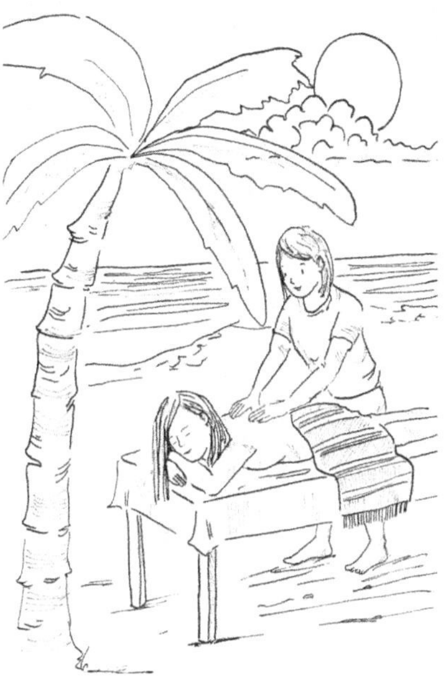

I love getting a massage! As soon as I lie down on a massage table, I can feel my heart rate decreasing, especially if it is a heated table—a special treat! On a daily basis, I love the feeling of using a cotton swab to dry and clean the outside portion of my ears after a shower. To me, this tactile sensation is worth the couple extra seconds it takes, and I keep an extra stash of cotton swabs just in case my kids use my regular supply for an art project and they disappear. I also simply enjoy the feeling of warm water on my skin in the shower. But picking up my hair that has fallen out while shampooing and throwing it away? Not so much. We don't need to make sense of or judge ourselves about which sensation we love. It doesn't have to make sense. Instead, I encourage you to purposely be present for some moments throughout your day and become more aware of your likes and dislikes of everyday sensations.

Do: Take a moment to absorb and become conscious of all the tactile information around you.
Reflect: What tactile sensations do you love?

Rate Your Preferences

If you could have a day full of just the right amount of each kind of sensation, how much tactile/touch information would you prefer? Where do your rate yourself on the preference scale for tactile information on the "My Sensory World" resource? Clothes are a really good clue here. If you look at what the clothing is made out of, notice if it has a tag, look for extra decorative seams, and feel the material more than you notice what it looks like, you may be closer to a one. For me, because my tactile system is pretty sensitive and I prefer less light-touch tactile information, I will not buy an item of clothing even if it is really cute and on sale if it is made out of wool, angora, or even cashmere. Those fabrics itch my skin and are not my ideal tactile sensations. They are not worth buying because I will never wear them.

Also think about interactions with other people as they apply to the tactile system. COVID definitely made it more socially appropriate to have all different kinds of greetings. Reflect on it: Are you a person who prefers a hug? Are you good with someone coming up behind you and giving you a hug unexpectedly? If so, you may be closer to **10**. If your preference is more along the lines of, "I'd love to wave to you from here," or maybe, depending on the day and person, you want to greet with an elbow tap or fist bump, maybe you're a little closer to a **1** on the tactile preference scale. Mark your ideal amount of tactile information.

Chapter 5

Your Current Reality

Now rate your reality on the "My Sensory World" resource. How much tactile information is in your routine day or week? I remember the too-much alarm going off when I was nursing my babies. It had been more nursing than not within a five-year period, and I was feeling the difference between my ideal amount of tactile information and my reality. I loved nursing my kids, but my tactile system was overloaded. It was a mismatch.

Are you cleaning up crumbs on the table or a dirty high-chair tray many times a day? Are you getting a lot of tactile information while cooking meals or riding a crowded bus? Do you make slime with your kids or play with Play-Doh daily? What clothes do you need to wear for your job? What type of fabric is your bedding, and whom do you share your bed with? Rate your typical amount of tactile information.

Your Current Reality

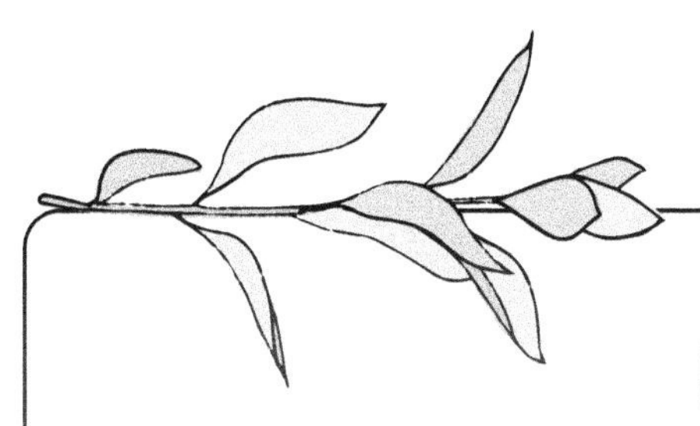

CHAPTER 6

Olfactory/Smell Sensation

"Smell is a potent wizard that transports you across thousands of miles and all the years you have lived."

- Helen Keller -

Our sense of smell or olfaction is also crucial to both survival and thriving. This sense starts developing around three weeks into development and is fully established at 28 to 30 weeks in utero! In your nose, you have 500 types of *smell detectors* (*odorant receptors*) perceiving scents and a couple million receptor cells. The cells activate in different combinations when little odor molecules bond to the receptors, detecting a trillion distinct smells. Scent molecules change the way receptors in the nose are activated in the future. The brain makes sense of smells through overlapping activation patterns, like computer coding or chords on the piano.

Limbic System: Deep in the brain, this area helps us process emotions, drives motivation and rewards, and makes new memories. The bridge between your brainstem (automatic control center for basic life functions) and the cerebral cortex (outer layer of the brain).

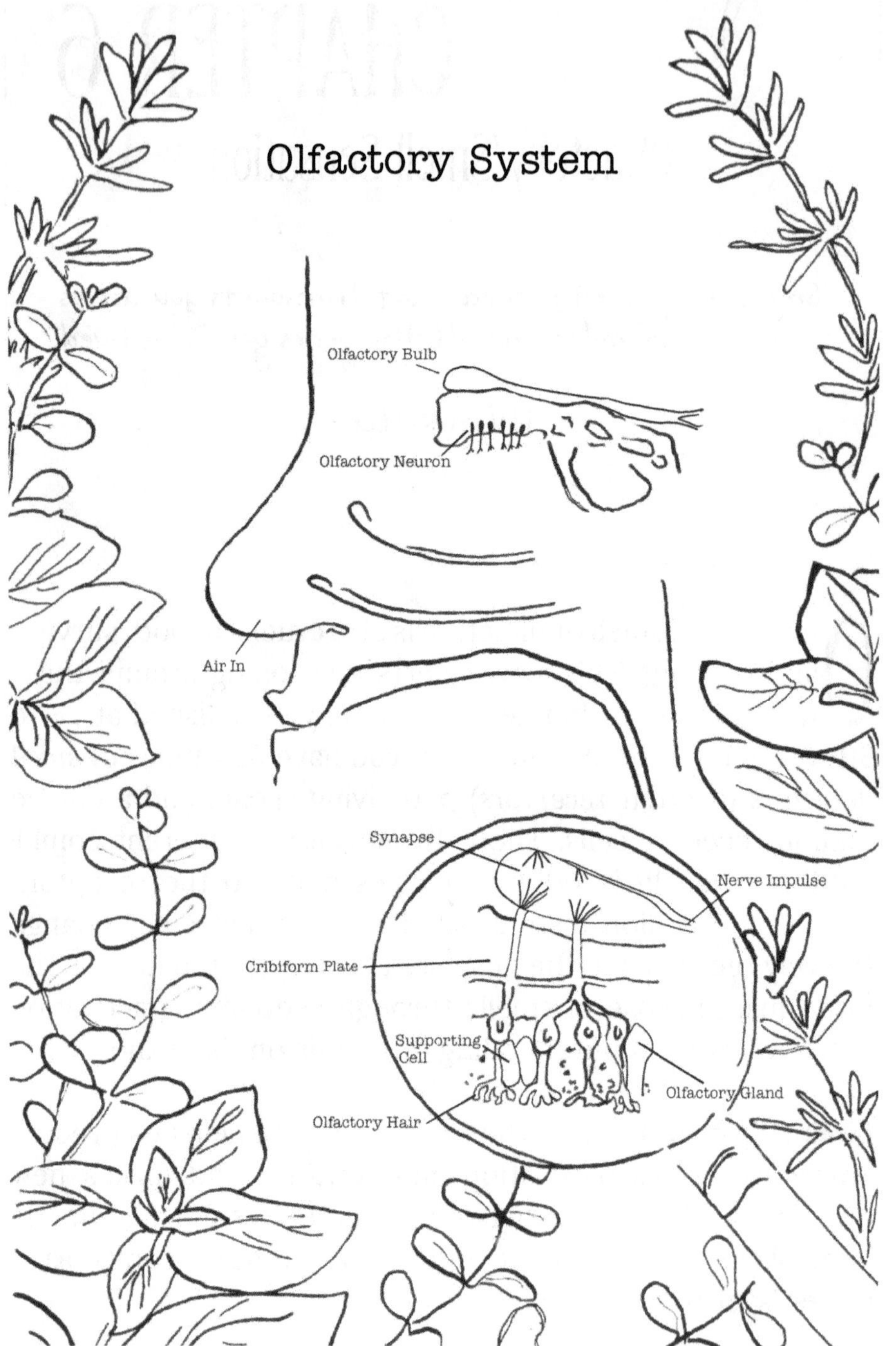
Olfactory System
Olfactory Bulb
Olfactory Neuron
Air In
Synapse
Nerve Impulse
Cribiform Plate
Supporting Cell
Olfactory Gland
Olfactory Hair

Chapter 6

The olfactory discrimination process is much more complex than the tactile system's additive, "You felt it here," and "You don't feel it here," process. A lovely morning cup of coffee can have 800 odor molecules! The sense of smell is as miraculous as it is mysterious, and the details of how scent detection works when multiple scents are mixed together puzzled scientists for a long time.

The power of smell comes from what happens next on the journey of the message to the brain. Smell messages do not go through the same pathway in the brain as other sense information, which goes to the *thalamus*, a sensory relay station (think train station), in the brain. Instead, olfactory information goes directly to the main areas in the brain that process smell like the Piriform cortex and your *limbic system*, which helps you feel emotions and make memories. A smell can trigger vivid, emotionally charged memories quickly and intensely, for good or bad. Fond memories evoked by smells impact regions of the brain and body, decreasing inflammation, improving memory recall, and increasing slower, deeper breathing. Your sense of smell can be an effective tool in your arsenal of regulation and wellness.

On a survival level, you need to quickly detect a propane leak so you can get out of the house safely. If the smell of smoke from an unplanned fire wafts toward you, your stress response can be activated unconsciously and help you escape danger.

On the other hand, smells can activate your calm response and bring a pleasant memory into your conscious awareness. For instance, the smell of lavender transports me back to a happy summer day with my kids giggling and dancing through a field of lavender with live music playing and a gorgeous sunset in the distance. Even on the hardest day, Earl Grey tea brewing brings my nervous system and heart back to my grandmother's house, where love comforts me when I'm feeling down.

Little side note here:

With this kind of powerful neurological circuitry wired in all of us, it is so important that we choose curiosity if someone around us has a sudden spike in emotion, heart rate, or grumpiness. Maybe they are smelling something that brings back a memory. If you choose to ask about it in a non-judgmental, open way, you may get to connect with them on a deeper level as they let you into a vulnerable place, an experience that was tucked away.

I realized the importance of this curiosity and openhearted approach with a family I worked with a while back. Absolutely beside himself, a father called me because, in the past year, his son, Greyson, had gotten kicked out of four preschools, was destroying their house, *and* was tearing their family apart. Baffled and frustrated, the teachers told Greyson's parents he would seem fine one moment and then suddenly push other preschoolers, throw things across the room, or start yelling. Greyson's little brother was scared of him. His parents were exhausted and so confused. They were fighting with each other: Did he need boundaries? Consequences? Attention?

Greyson came to the clinic one day, and we started playing various games with different sensations. As I pulled out the scented markers, I noticed his eyes getting big, his cheeks getting flushed, and him turning his body away from the table. I proceeded to draw an ocean on my piece of paper with caution and curiosity. A lot of four- and five-year-olds don't love drawing or writing letters, but this seemed like a more significant response than not preferring an activity. As the blueberry scent of the blue marker spread, he forcefully slid the markers across the table and yelled, "No more!" Seconds later, I heard his dysregulation loud and clear as he threw up all over the table. He did not purposely throw up in an act of defiance. He was not trying to make me have a bad day. What had happened?

After cleaning up and playing on the rock wall in our sensory gym (with the scented markers put away), we wrapped up the evaluation on a positive note. I called his parents later that afternoon to check in. When I mentioned his strong, negative response to the scented markers, they gasped. They revealed that Greyson had been abused by an extended family member at a fourth of July gathering right after eating a blueberry-and-strawberry dessert. So terrible! Now it all made sense. Over time, we worked together to start understanding the smells that brought his nervous system back to that traumatic event.

Learning about how past sensory pairings impacted his present experiences guided our plan for how to respond at home and at school. His pushing, yelling, and throwing were not a need for discipline. Greyson needed help. Help started with understanding sensation.

***Sensory pairings*:** Also known as *emotional associations*, are when an event happens at the same time or close to an event, linking sensations to an emotion in our brains.

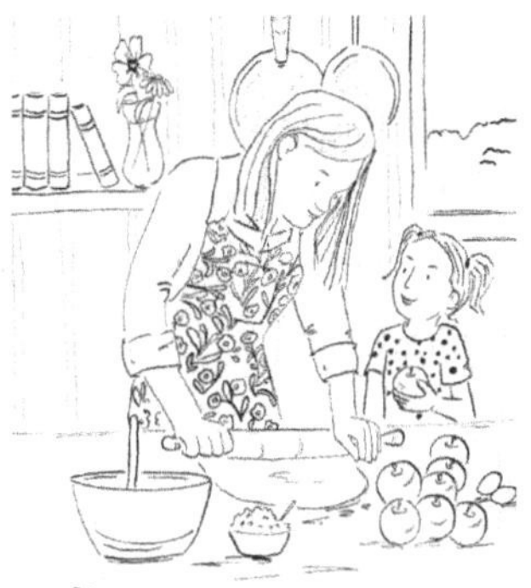

Back to the sense of smell, what are your favorite scents? I love the smell of my mom's apple pie baking in the fall and gingerbread in the oven around Christmas, a breeze blowing over freshly mown grass in the early summer and grilling meat and veggies on summer evenings. The fresh smell after a rain delights my smell receptors. And the smell of my morning coffee brewing because I got it ready and on a timer the night before helps me get up in the morning, even when I am still so tired after a busy couple of days or months.

Do: Take a moment to absorb and become conscious of all the olfactory information around you.
Reflect: What olfactory sensations do you love?

Rate Your Preferences

As far as your ideal level of smell information goes, what is your sensory preference? Of course, it varies based on what kind of scents we are talking about. You may be closer to a **10** on our scale of olfactory preference if you are a person who has 20 different kinds of perfumes, and not only do you vary which one you use, but you also mix and match, creating your own perfume amazingness. And then you may be closer to the **1** side if you buy everything unscented or even make your own deodorant and soap, eliminating all fragrances.

I started to consciously notice my preference being more on the **1** side when I was pregnant and wanting fewer and milder scents around me. When I flew on Southwest Airlines, which did not assign seats, I didn't choose my seat based on what a person looked like, how big they were, or anything like that. I was smelling my way down the aisle, trying to decide if I would be able to handle the olfactory environment around me for the whole flight.

Record your preference rating on the "My Sensory World" resource.

Your Current Reality

And on the sensory reality side, smell your way through a normal day. How much olfactory information is a part of your regular routine? As I write this book, I have so many flowers blooming in my garden, and fresh bouquets of stock and lilies fill my living room area. I have my favorite lavender hand cream that I typically put on during my first meeting of the day. I don't have any air fresheners in my car, but some days my kids' leftover food adds an interesting smell to the dropping-off-the-kids part of the day. My shampoo and conditioner are mildly scented, and the laundry detergent is unscented. No more diapers to change, and my kids clean their own shared bathroom. When we are not out and about, the fragrances of cooking fill the house around dinner time. So, my olfactory score for real life is pretty close to my ideal amount of scent information.

What's your rating of your typical amount and intensity of olfactory information?

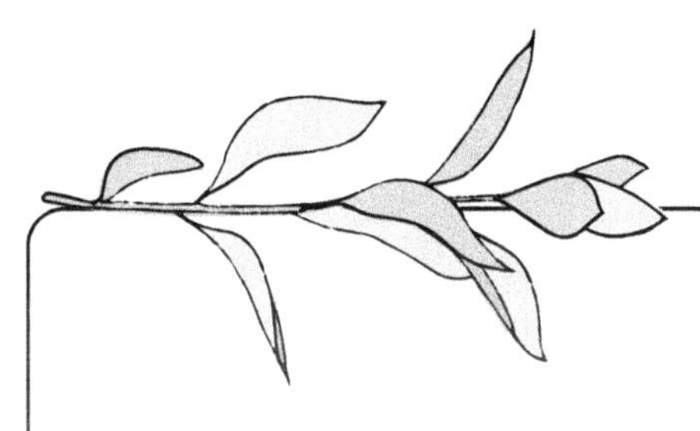

CHAPTER 7

Gustatory/Taste Sensation

"All you need is love. But a little chocolate now and then doesn't hurt."

- Charles M. Schulz -

Let's explore taste sensation! The gustatory (taste) system is a fun sense to think about from a regulation and energy level perspective. We often think about food as nutrition, a time-consuming fact of life for caregivers of young children who are constantly feeding growing little ones, a battle of calories and yum, or a foodie adventure of fun flavor. We can also eat something sour to wake us up. People eat comfort food to connect them to a fond memory. How about intentionally crunching on some carrots to chill after an intense meeting or drinking a thick smoothie while working on a hard project to help focus?

Let's start with the development of the gustatory system. Your taste receptors start developing around seven to eight weeks *in utero*, and the salty receptors develop last, at around four months old. Your taste buds come in five varieties: sweet, salty, bitter, umami, and sour. Complex flavors are perceived in the brain by activating different combinations of these and with the help of the olfactory system. The receptors for taste decrease in number, size, and capability after the age of 40.

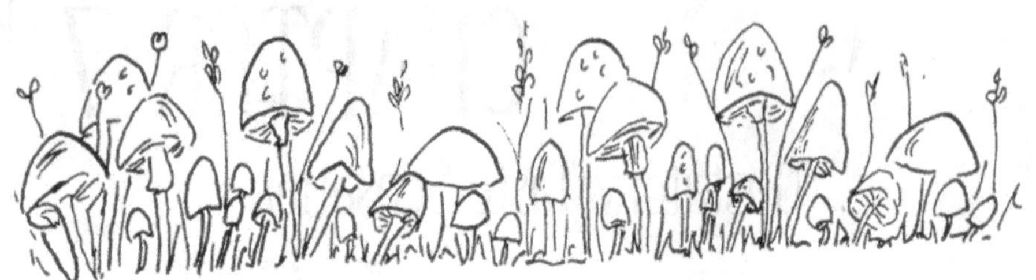

Gustatory System

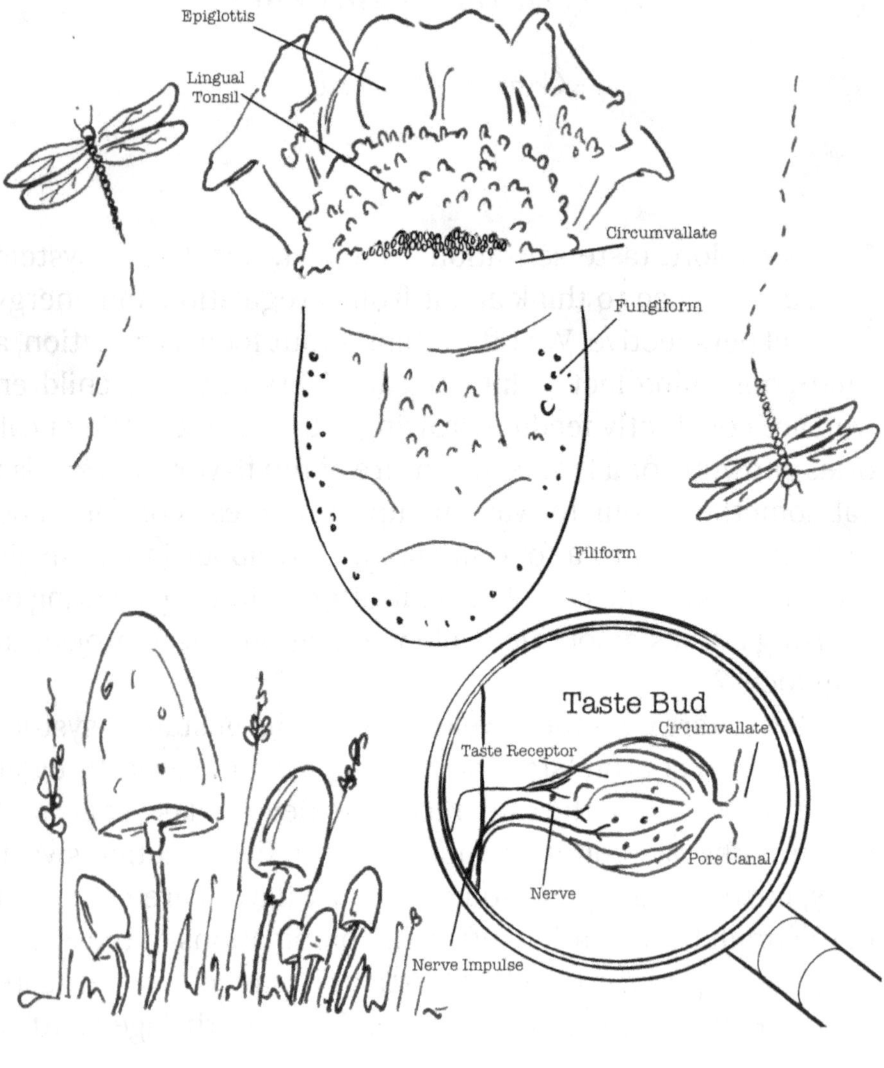

Epiglottis
Lingual Tonsil
Circumvallate
Fungiform
Filiform

Taste Bud
Circumvallate
Taste Receptor
Pore Canal
Nerve
Nerve Impulse

Chapter 7

So many wonderful flavors come to mind when I take a deep breath and reflect on what I love! When I'm busy, though, I forget to make time for eating flavorful, exciting food. I love tomatillo salsa with chips, frozen bananas with chocolate and peanut butter on top, spring rolls with spicy peanut sauce, and fresh chocolate chip cookies! When life gets hard and the reality of the out-of-control-ness of the world feels heavy, taking a moment to eat something you love and direct all your attention to the different sensations as you eat it can be the mini-vacation you need, in your own home or office. Fully present, mindful eating, even just for five minutes, can work wonders. Tuning into the textures, smells, and tastes of what you are eating is the opposite of eating to numb the pain or push away feelings.

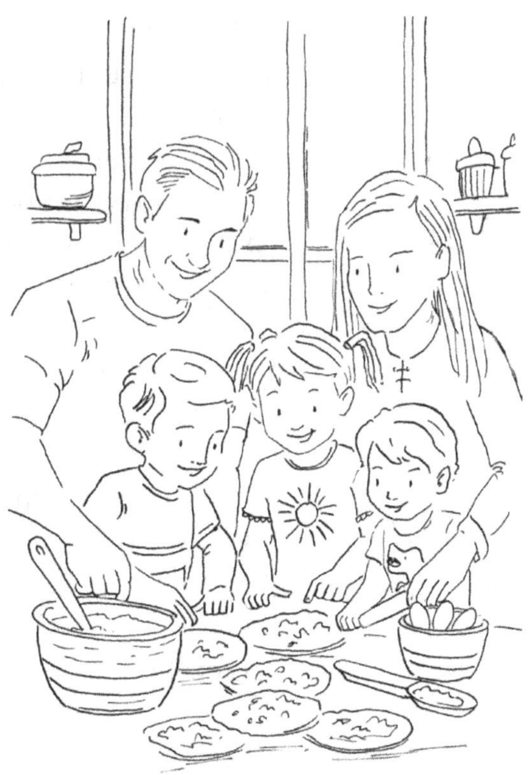

Do: Take a moment to absorb and become conscious of any taste information you are perceiving.

Try this: Next time something tastes a bit bland (whether it is because you are getting older or not), try adding lemon juice instead of salt. Lemon increases the flavor and can trick your taste buds into thinking it is more salty and yummy without the negative side effects of too much salt.

Reflect: What taste sensations do you love?

Rate Your Preferences

So, from an ideal sensory level perspective, how much taste sensation do you prefer? Are you a person who cooks with a whole bunch of different spices? I'm not necessarily talking about the spicy, hotness level of the spices you use, but the variety and number of seasonings you use if you prepare food just for yourself. The more you prefer, the closer to a **10** you are. On the opposite extreme, if you prefer one brand of plain crackers and one brand of chicken nuggets dipped in a simple sauce, you are likely closer to a **1**. Remember, no answer is a wrong or right answer here. No number on the scale is better than another. Gently remind yourself that you don't need to "should" yourself about this, saying, "I should like more flavor." Or, "I shouldn't like all that spice." It is all about bringing awareness to your preferences in this season of life: a different kind of knowing and loving yourself. It's about noticing, right? And *then* using sensation as a tool. When I have a strong peppermint in my mouth, I'm more alert to drive late at night. More to come on that front!

Rate your level of taste preference on the "My Sensory World" resource.

Chapter 7

Your Current Reality

Taste is an area where, depending on what part of raising kids or taking care of parents you are in, you may discover a big difference between your ideal sensation and your daily life. The reality of doing daily life with others can be hard in the gustatory area because of strong preference differences. You may be imagining a beautiful, seared fish with chimichurri sauce and an exciting side salad with all sorts of rare veggies, but your partner or kids want nothing to do with it! They were looking forward to a quesadilla with one kind of cheese or boxed mac and cheese. Preparing two meals is exhausting, and over time the meals on regular rotation evolve to work for everyone, potentially leaving you far away from what you want to eat. So take a moment to consider, what is your rating of your typical amount of taste sensation? Keep on recording these on your "My Sensory World" resource. We will be using these ratings later.

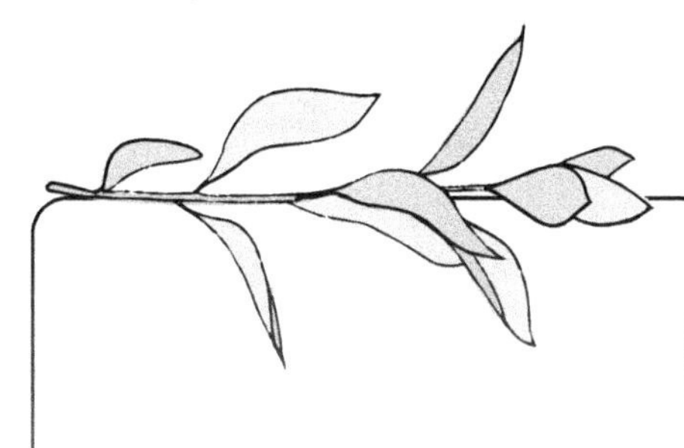

CHAPTER 8

Proprioceptive/Muscles Sensation

"In every walk with nature one receives far more than he seeks."

- John Muir -

Proprio what? Elementary school and even high school anatomy and physiology don't often cover the next two senses. But the proprioceptive and vestibular (coming next) senses are superpower senses, foundational to who you are as a person and how you interact with the world, and crucial to your growth in sensory wellness.

Proprioception is your awareness of your body's position: how much your muscles are contracted. This sense guides the movement of your arms and legs without having to look. I use proprioceptive information to pick up my cup and drink some coffee without pouring it all over myself. I can feel the weight of the cup, determine how much liquid is in the cup, and perceive how much and how fast my muscles are contracting or extending to move the cup with accuracy—all automatically and unconsciously!

When I work with people with sensory integration and processing challenges, I have them do a little game I call *reindeer antlers*. Try this: Put your hands above your head where a

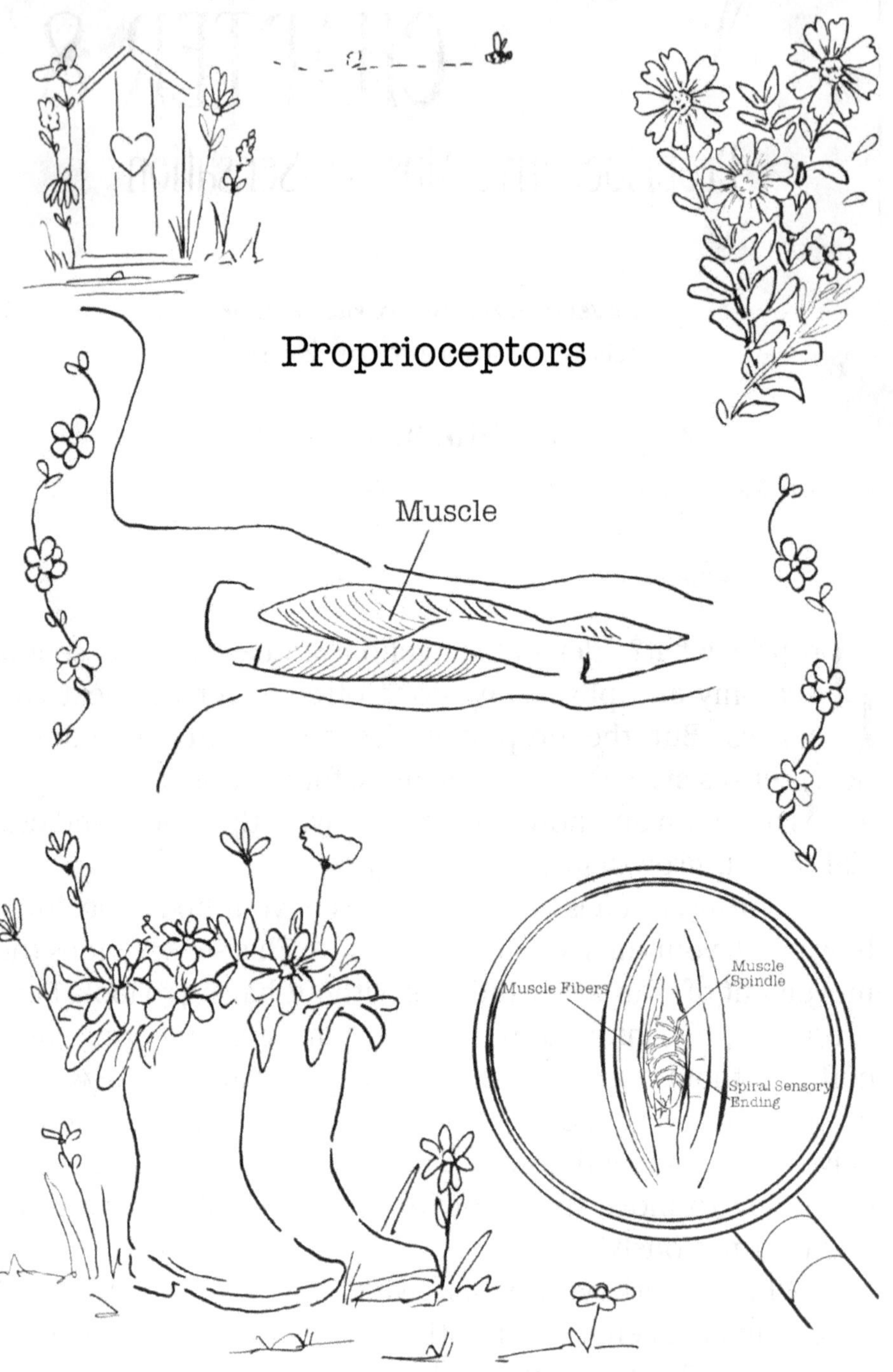
Proprioceptors
Muscle
Muscle Fibers
Muscle Spindle
Spiral Sensory Ending

reindeer would have its antlers. Now change your hand position from five fingers all straight to making a number one sign or cross your index and middle fingers. You didn't have to look at your hands to know if your hand position was correct, right?

Proprioceptive receptors are in all of your muscle fibers and joints and deep in your skin. When you get a massage or chew a piece of gum, you are increasing your proprioceptive input and, in turn, increased serotonin, dopamine, and oxytocin (happy, feel-good neurotransmitters) are released in your brain. Serotonin is the same neurotransmitter that becomes more available when someone struggling with depression or anxiety takes an SSRI (selective serotonin reuptake inhibitors) antidepressant. *I'm not saying replace an antidepressant if you have been advised by a medical professional to take one.* What I am saying is that when you exercise and contract your muscles or chew on something like beef jerky or those big, crunchy pretzels, it really makes your jaw work, and the muscle contraction can improve your mood using the same mechanisms as an antidepressant. Proprioceptive input also increases the calm response that goes with increased activation of the parasympathetic nervous system, supporting our regulation and ability to intentionally and kindly respond to daily events.

Proprioception starts developing early, around seven weeks *in utero*, and then it keeps going longer into development than any of the other senses, wrapping up around age 18. New drivers out on the road, with their proprioceptive systems not quite fully developed, really need to hold the wheel with both hands and not to hold a cell phone while driving, for this and other reasons.

I love proprioceptive input! I love sleeping with my cozy, weighted blanket. The best way to start my day, if I'm not paddling out to surf during the sunrise, is lifting weights and doing my favorite cardio: the Versaclimber, a whole body workout where you move your arms and legs like you are climbing a mountain. I feel strong and grounded, ready to flex with whatever life brings. Swimming is also high on my list of favorites, moving through the water, weightless and free.

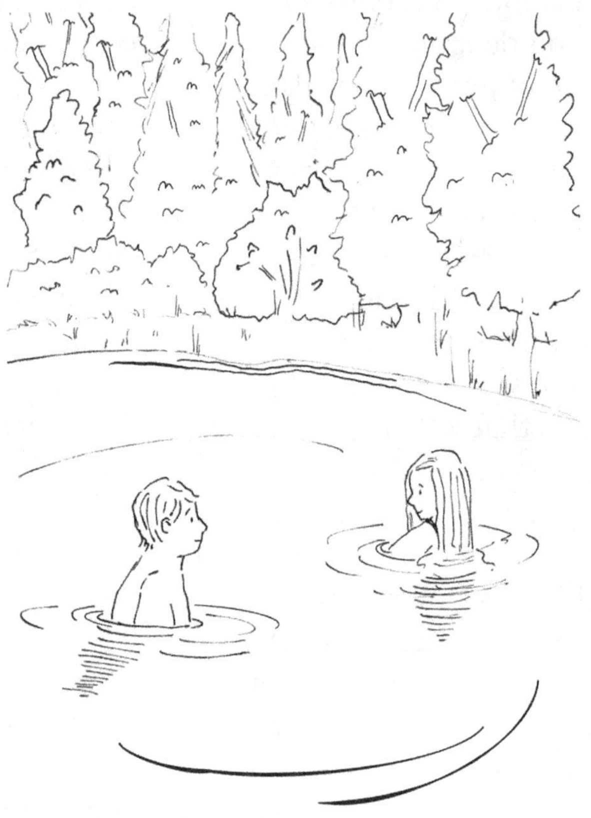

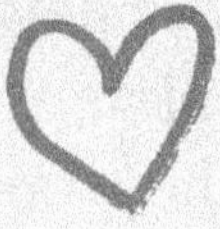

Do: Take a moment to absorb and become conscious of all the proprioceptive information coming up to your brain. Which muscles are contracting? How are you breathing: deep into your stomach or more in your chest? Through your nose or through your mouth? Are you chewing on anything right now?

Reflect: What proprioceptive sensations do you love?

Rate Your Preferences

Now for your ideal sensory lifestyle: How much proprioceptive information would you prefer? If you are a person who loves massages, regularly walks with friends and takes Pilates classes, and enjoys cuddling while watching a movie, you may be closer to a **10**. Are you constantly chewing gum or something crunchy? That could be an indicator of a higher rating too. If you're a person who feels more partial to sitting and reading a book than going to yoga, you may be closer to a **1**. Rate your level of proprioceptive preference on the "My Sensory World" resource.

Your Current Reality

And reality: How much proprioceptive information is a part of your regular routine right now? Are you working out regularly? Chewing on ice while working on a project? Mostly sitting in front of a computer? Sitting on a large exercise ball? Driving a car around most of the day to get kids where they need to be? Driving includes a little contraction of your calf muscles, some posture muscles, and arm muscles, but not a ton of proprioceptive input. Do you have a weighted blanket on your bed? Mark your level of your typical proprioceptive input. Start noticing how close or far apart your ideal mark for proprioception is from your current reality of proprioceptive input.

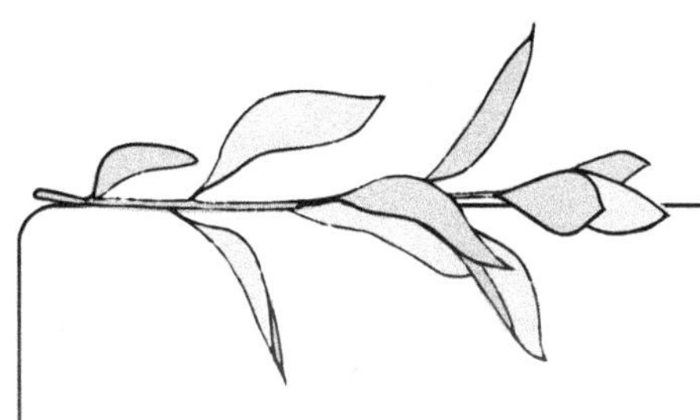

CHAPTER 9

Vestibular/Movement Sensation

"All that is important is this one moment in movement. Make the moment important, vital, and worth living. Do not let it slip away unnoticed and unused."

- Martha Graham -

"When I experience joy, it feels like it all builds up within me and breathes life into my limbs. I feel and express joy... in the way I move and interact with the space around me."

- Mailani McKelvy (autistic creator) -

Another sense you don't often learn about in school, the *vestibular (movement and balance) sense*, tells you about how your body is moving: up and down, side to side, forward and backward, and all the combinations possible. Vestibular information also grounds you quite literally, telling you about how gravity is impacting you. Knowing where you stand in relation to the surface of the earth is crucial. Movement information also provides the foundation for balance. The receptors for the vestibular system are right next to your auditory receptors in the inner ear and include the *utricle*, *saccule*, and the *semicircular canals*. Vestibular information generates

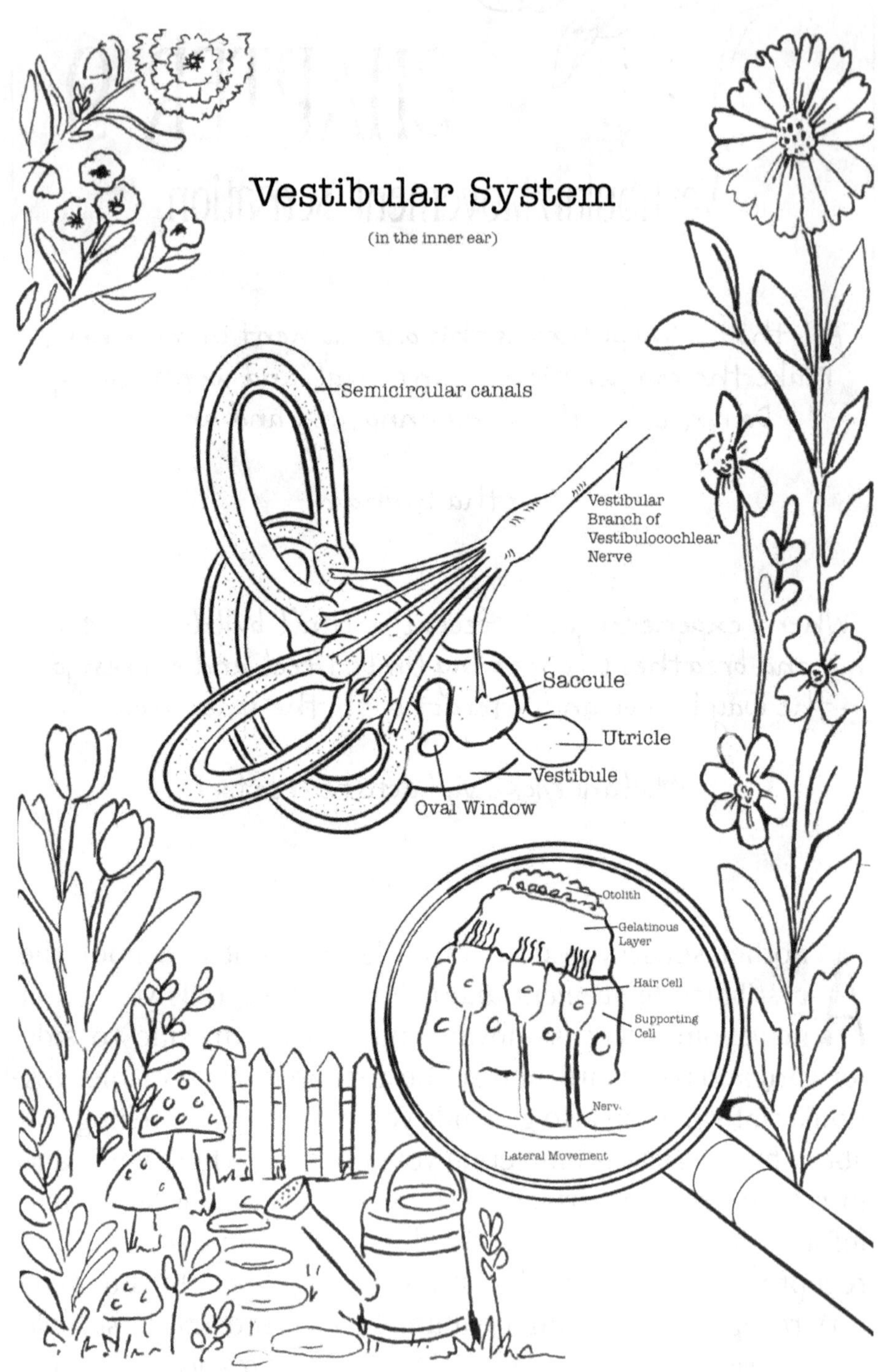

Vestibular System
(in the inner ear)
Semicircular canals
Vestibular Branch of Vestibulocochlear Nerve
Saccule
Utricle
Vestibule
Oval Window
Otolith
Gelatinous Layer
Hair Cell
Supporting Cell
Nerv
Lateral Movement

unconscious complex math equations using a three-dimensional x, y, and z axis to tell you about how you are moving in relation to people and objects in the space around you. Are you going to bump into the branch on the trail ahead? The fluid in the semicircular canals (think enclosed water slides at a water park) moves and pushes over hair cells that send the brain information, so you know if you are speeding up or slowing down and in which direction you are moving.

We can stay calm when walking toward someone because we can tell from their body language and also from this unconscious math equation going on in the background if they are going to crash into us football-tackle style, or if we are on track for a gentle hug.

Try this: stand up and spin around a couple of times. Or if you are sitting in an office chair, stay seated and spin around. When you stop, count how many seconds you feel dizzy. If that sounds like a bad idea or if you get vertigo easily, try just tilting your head up and looking at the ceiling and then back down at the ground multiple times. What do you notice? That is your vestibular system.

The vestibular system starts developing around day 33 in the womb and is established and connected by the fifth month of development: the earliest system to be well developed! The vestibular system is fully mature by age 15, just in time to get a driver's permit in a lot of the United States.

I have had a bit of a love/hate or slow-to-warm-up-to relationship with vestibular information. As a kid, I remember going to the county fair on a swelteringly hot day. I was showing rabbits in the agricultural area, and we got a free wristband to go on all the rides. My younger sisters were excited about the rides, but I immediately started feeling sick to my stomach. We started with a "little kid" ride that looked like a black spider, with each of the legs having a spinner at the end with seats for a couple of kids. Hesitantly, I said I would go on it, but as we waited in line, I started to have second thoughts. With sweat dripping down my back from both the heat and my nerves, I climbed up, and the attendant checked my seat belt. Satisfied that we were all strapped in, he turned the ride on, and I felt the acceleration. We started spinning as the spider legs went up and down. Bad idea! I closed my eyes, but it didn't matter. Tears were streaming down my face and flying toward my sister in the seat next to me. I was about to be sick when our turn was over. The spider came to a stop, but I felt nauseous the rest of the day. Not fun.

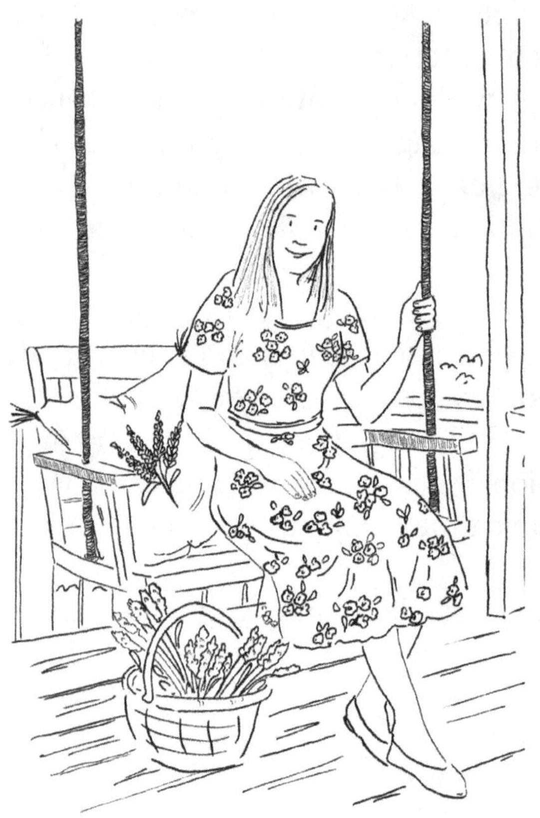

Over time, I have worked on adjusting the way I take in movement information because I want to enjoy some basic rides with my kids and improve my surfing. I recently celebrated with my youngest son when I kept my eyes open the whole time on a ride at Disney World and didn't feel sick at all! I still pass on the spinning teacups though. I do love the gentler vestibular sensations of swinging on a porch swing and riding a wave in the ocean, moving up and down the face of the wave ahead of the crashing white water.

Do: Take a moment to be aware of any of the vestibular information you are registering right now. Are you listening to this book while going on a walk? Are you lying in a hammock while reading this?
Reflect: What vestibular sensations do you love?

Rate Your Preferences

Movement-wise, would your favorite day be an amusement park where there were no lines on any ride and you could just enjoy them over and over and over again? Then maybe you rate yourself a **10** on this ideal vestibular sensation scale? How do you like water slides? Flips in the pool? On the other hand, if, when you move from sitting up to lying down or from lying down to sitting up, you get a little dizzy and it's not your favorite thing to do, you are probably closer to a **1** here. Maybe riding a bike or swinging is not what you choose on a free weekend. How much movement do you want? Make sure to record your rating.

Your Current Reality

And now shifting gears, what does your vestibular reality look like during a typical week? Are you running around, chasing five-year-olds at soccer practice because you are helping coach? Are you sitting in front of a computer most of the day, or driving a lot? Are you in an acrobatic club? Go ziplining every weekend? Rate the amount of movement information that is part of your regular routine. Remember, for vestibular receptors to be activated, your head position needs to change, like the little dot moving on a map app on your phone. Record this one too.

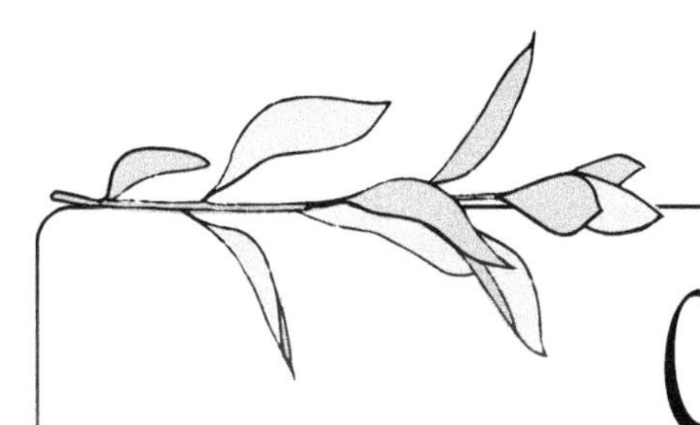

CHAPTER 10

Visceral Interoceptive/ Internal Organs Sensation

"The body has its own language. Listen to the whispers before they become screams."

- Unknown, contemporary proverb -

"My interoception awareness is a mix of under responsive in some areas, over responsive in others—and an overarching inability to differentiate or understand many of my body signals."

- Dr. Megan Anna Neff, autistic psychologist -

Sense data also comes into your brain from your internal organs, telling you if you are full, hungry, thirsty, or need to go to the bathroom. This visceral interoceptive information comes from your heart, lungs, digestive system, and other organs. While research about the timeline of development of this part of your nervous system is on-going, we know visceral interoception develops continuously and throughout life. This type of interoceptive input is key for physical health, emotional memory, learning, and decision making.

Visceral Interoception

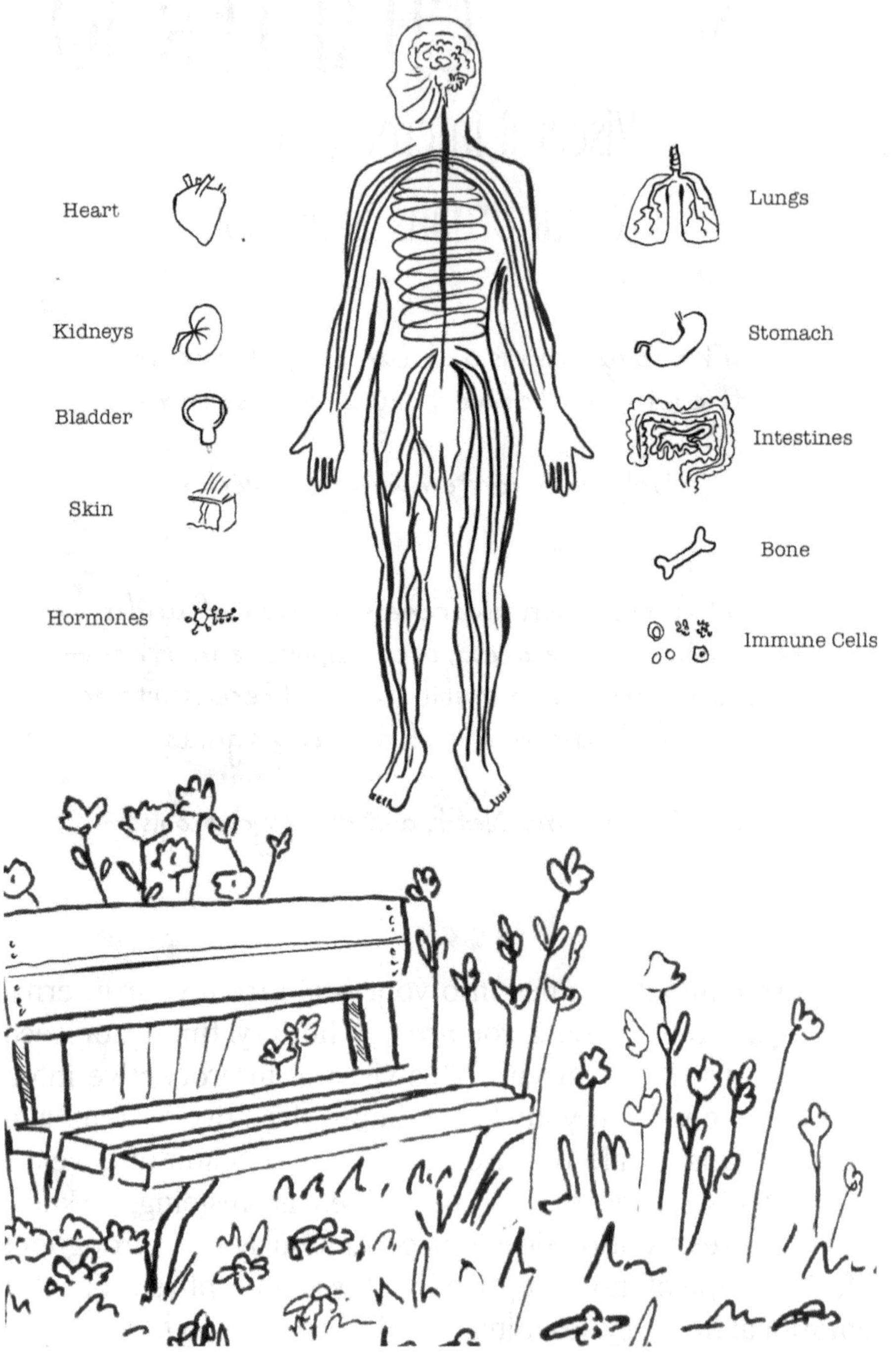

What are these interoceptor receptors like? It depends on which organ in your body we are talking about. Approximately 40,000 neurons make up a version of a brain within your heart: an intricate network of several types of neurons, neurotransmitters, proteins, and support cells like those found in the brain in your head. The heart brain acts independently of the cranial brain: learning, remembering, and even feeling and sensing! Your *enteric nervous system* (the complex network of nerves throughout your digestive system that manages digestion of food without input from your brain) is 200 to 600,000,000 neurons: another brain-like system in your intestines! For comparison, that is two-thirds the size of a cat's nervous system in your digestive system, and your own cranial brain is only about 80,000,000,000 neurons big!

Insular Cortex: An area deep in the middle of your brain that integrates internal body sensations and sensory information in the environment with emotions, thoughts, and actions. The insular cortex alerts you when you are hungry or full, or feel anxious, or perceive pain. Playing a crucial role in having empathy and self-awareness, this area of your brain supports your development of your sense of self and integration of information for intentional decision making.

Anterior Cingulate Cortex: In the front of the brain on the inner wall of each side, this area helps you manage attention, emotions, and actions. The anterior cingulate cortex is actively supporting when you express and regulate emotions, weigh out different options while making a tricky decision, learn from your mistakes and navigate a conflict.

Have you ever had a "gut feeling" about something? Your gut can be very smart. It is wise to pause and take those feelings into consideration. Interoceptive information is crucial for processing emotions and activates your *salience network* (your priority filter, see appendix for more information on brain networks) with increased activity in specific parts of the brain (specifically the *insular cortex* and the *anterior cingulate cortex*). Emotions activate areas all over your brain, like a beautiful blossoming flower with the stem set right in the insular cortex (my current favorite part of the brain) and the roots spread all over your body stretching down to sensory receptors. The nervous system activation during emotion forms an hourglass shape throughout your body and brain.

Interoception guides the experience and interpretation of emotions. People with better interoceptive accuracy are more likely to experience emotions more vividly. We need to be able to recognize anxiety, anger, or overwhelm rising up in us so we can consciously decide what we want to do about the emotion. Interoception is a core component of emotional intelligence.

Who doesn't want to feel more joy today than yesterday? As Brené Brown has shown in her research, it doesn't work to shut out one emotion and still feel others. One of my favorite sayings is, "Feelings are much like waves. We can't stop them from coming, but we can choose which one to surf," by Jonatan Mårtensson. Interoceptive awareness is the key to choosing our waves.

On the other hand, decreased interoceptive awareness can lead to poor decision making and is correlated with eating disorders and post-traumatic stress disorder (PTSD). Often, to help a person survive after a traumatic experience, the person's interoceptive system may turn off or may become unhelpfully loud, overwhelming their brain and impacting the person's ability to do what they love. Low interoceptive sensitivity is linked to increased anxiety, depression, and panic disorder. People with ADHD and autism may have reduced interoceptive accuracy, which leads to difficulties with noticing bodily cues that inform emotion interpretation. The visceral, internal organ component of interoceptive information is imperative for overall wellness.

Interoceptive sensation is more complicated than the turn-it-up-or-down nature of the other senses we have talked about. You can still think about what kinds of interoceptive information you love. After some health challenges that resulted in my not being hungry often, I have come to really appreciate the sensation of feeling hungry. I'm not sure *love* is the right way of describing it, but hunger messages are reassuring, telling me my body is working. One type of interoceptive input I definitely love? Orgasms! Shown in the literature to be important for overall well-being of all people, life satisfaction, and psychological and physical functioning, we don't need science to tell us orgasms are wonderful.

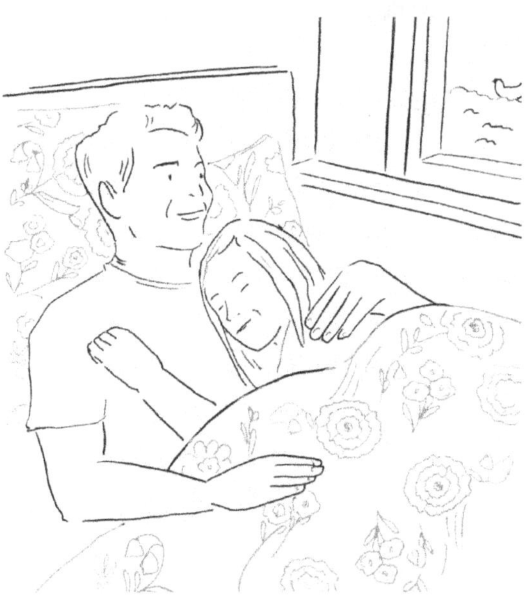

Research confirms and explains that the *noticing* component of interoception predicts frequency of orgasm by yourself and with a partner, *attention regulation* predicts greater frequency and satisfaction of solitary orgasms, and *body trusting* predicts orgasm satisfaction both during masturbation and during intimacy with another! These components of interoception are delineated on the Multidimensional Assessment of Interoceptive Awareness (MAIA) developed by Wolf E. Mehling, MD, and colleagues at the University of California, San Francisco (2018). If you would like to explore these components of interoception further, this resource is in the public domain and available to use for free! Orgasms also increase parasympathetic activation, helping us ebb and flow with life stressors and improving heart rate variability.

Do: Take a moment to become aware of any messages your internal body sensory receptors are sending you right now. Can you feel your heartbeat?
Reflect: What visceral interoceptive sensations do you love?

Rate Your Preferences

We need to approach this a little differently from the way we look at other senses, where it made more sense to think about ideal amounts and your routine amounts of input. However, valuable insights may come to light upon reflecting on your perception of this internal sensory information. Your awareness of interoceptive processing may not match your needs, and it can be adjusted, with the support of a loving community and often mental health professionals. So reflect for a moment on how much awareness of your internal messages from your body you would prefer. You will rate yourself closer to a **10** if you want to notice often how full your bladder is, your hunger level, pain in different body parts, and other internal sensations. If you would rather not often hear these or other messages from within your body, rate yourself closer to a **1**. I find myself somewhere in the middle on this one in this season of my sensational life. I don't really want to hear every time my knees are aching, but I do want to keep tabs on how my overall inflammation is doing. I'd rather not need to go to the bathroom as often, and I do feel gratitude for still being aware of how badly I need to go, ideally before I sneeze. I want to lean into and continue learning more about what sensations move my body closer to orgasm and how fast, so I'd prefer to stay on the more side of the continuum there. I also find reassurance in feeling my heartbeat and tuning into my breathing, like checking in with an old friend. So where do you rate your preference for internal sensations?

Your Current Reality

Let's talk about a typical day in the area of interoceptive information from your organs. Do you hear messages from your internal organs? Do you consciously notice your heart beat? Do you perceive messages about hunger? If loudly and often, you may be closer to a **10** on the current reality rating. Do you feel the need to use the bathroom only once it becomes almost an emergency and is painful? You may be closer to a **1**. Go ahead and fill in the last rating on your "My Sensory World" resource.

A quick side note here: Sometimes, tuning into your internal sensations can be lifesaving. If you find yourself noticing things in your body that don't seem right, I encourage you to check in with a medical professional. And if you don't have a medical professional that you feel comfortable sharing this information with, do your best to find one. If necessary, advocate for a change! I know how hard the process of finding a medical professional that aligns with your approach to health and wellness can be, and it is worth it. Find professionals you trust. Give it your all. You are worth it and you've got a lot of sensational living to do!

Noticing Your Thoughts

As we wrap up this section on deepening our understanding and awareness of the senses and prepare to explore how to purposely use sensation to support our regulation and improve our life participation and satisfaction, take a moment to notice your thoughts about your thoughts (*metacognition*). Metacognition can reveal our self-compassion and kindness or lack thereof. As I have coached therapists and other professionals through taking care of themselves and tuning into their bodies, many people have told me this work revealed they were mean to themselves in ways they would never be to the people around them. I want to encourage you to set down self-judgment and ask yourself to stop saying any harsh words you are telling yourself. Be on the journey, a process we are all in as long as we have breath in our lungs. Some days you will feel like a rock star, and other days you will feel like a complete mess. It is okay. You are in good company.

Locus of control: The extent to which individuals believe they have control over the events of their lives, a concept developed by Julian Rotter, behaviorist.

Internal locus of control: Belief that you have a significant degree of control over your life and the outcome of situations.

Chapter 10

External locus of control: Belief that your life is largely controlled by external forces beyond your influence.

When you think about where your mind goes, do you notice any thoughts that sound like you are a victim, explaining your current reality in an "I'm stuck because" way? Sometimes people get stuck in a victim mentality state where they experience life as a series of events that are happening to them, where they feel they have no agency or power to change what is happening. Recounting their day could sound like, "The plumber ripped me off, a so-called friend blamed me for something I didn't do, and then, on the way here, two cars cut me off—reckless drivers everywhere!" Everyone has moments like these, but life is not enjoyable if every moment, every day, every year feels like a series of victim moments. If you have had "big T" traumas in your life like a horrific event or "little t" traumas like your senses intensely responding to life experiences daily, you may be more likely to shift into a victim mentality because your nervous system has been hijacked by trauma. A way of shifting out of a victim mentality is adjusting the various kinds of sensation. *Sense of agency* or an *internal locus of control* comes from increased interoceptive and exteroceptive sensory awareness and introspection. I can shift what's happening in my world to have a better day, regardless of what other people are doing, because I have the power of sensation.

"As water reflects the face,
so one's life reflects the heart."

- Proverbs 27:19 -

My Sensory World Reflections

Bring back out your "My Sensory World" resource. Look at the difference between your ideal amount and intensity of each type of sensation and your current amount of that type of sensory input on a regular basis.

- ✦ Which sense is the closest to having the same preference and reality rating?
- ✦ Which sense is the furthest from having the same preference and reality rating?
- ✦ Are there any shifts in your typical routine you want to make sooner than later?

We will continue reflecting on this together throughout section three.

SECTION 3

Multisensory Flourishing!

"Life is tough my darling, but so are you."

- Stephanie Bennett-Henry -

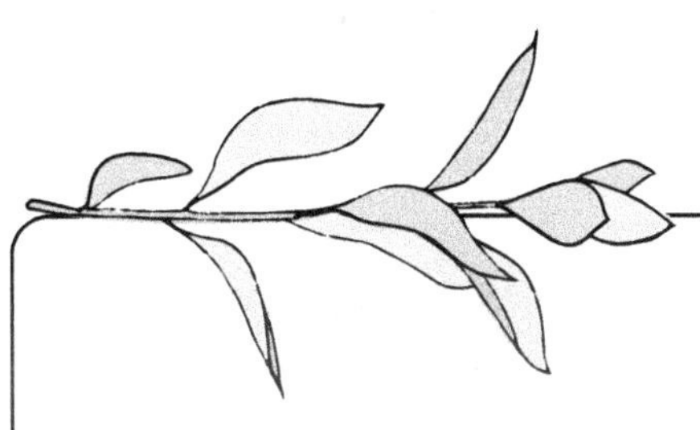

CHAPTER 11

Daily Energy Awareness

"Passion is energy. Feel the power that comes from focusing on what excites you."

- Oprah Winfrey -

How ready are you to do what you need to do today? Or even just the next thing on your schedule? Having the energy you need to do the next thing is based on how sensation impacts your alertness, level of distraction, and stress. Formally, energy and alertness are referred to as your *regulation arousal level.* This is different from sexual arousal, although the two can absolutely impact each other. The stress and calm responses we talked about earlier impact your regulation arousal level, as do many other aspects of life.

For instance:

- ✦ How did you sleep last night?
- ✦ What did you eat today?
- ✦ What thoughts are swirling around your head?
- ✦ What is on your To-Do list for the day?
- ✦ What deadlines do you have coming up?
- ✦ How did interactions go with people at work? At home?

What is the ideal energy level for what you have coming up next in your day? Higher arousal is not always better. It depends on the activity! No level of energy is inherently bad and, in certain circumstances, you benefit from being at every level. Your optimal performance or being your best self for a test, interview, or challenging interaction likely occurs in a middle zone of energy and alertness. When you are not about to fall asleep or feel so nervous you may throw up any minute, a middle zone of energy supports tapping into all your skills for a presentation at work.

I want to be at low energy when trying to fall asleep and stay asleep at night. If my car starts making strange noises while driving, I want higher arousal to command my attention so I can safely pull over and vigilantly determine my next steps. For me, a perfect application of energy level matching the event is going to experience live music. Part of my enjoyment can be the rush of adrenaline increasing my energy level as I see my favorite artist performing in concert. And sometimes, I love the low energy level that matches lying on the grass and listening to some blues, relaxed and chill.

Increasing your awareness of your energy level:

Do: Check in with your body. What energy level are you currently at: low, middle, high?

Reflect: What energy level would be ideal for what you are about to do next in your day? Do your current and needed energy levels match?

Some activities have a wider range of ideal energy level that will work, and the range is different for each person and in each season of life. A first-time parent starting to feed their little one solid food for the first time is likely going to need to be pretty dialed in to the middle of the curve. On the other hand, a caregiver who has helped many, many toddlers learn about new foods does not need to be as focused and centered as the new parent. The seasoned caregiver could be very tired or stressed and, in either case, be doing a safe and supportive job of feeding the little one.

Think about the first time you drove on your own after getting your driver's license! You needed to be very dialed in, and if you freaked out too much or felt too tired or distracted, you could have easily gotten in an accident. Now that you have driven more, hopefully you can safely drive within a pretty big range of energy levels.

Also, some people have a smaller range of energy levels that works for them to do what they need to do. Have you known anyone who seems fine one minute and then not so fine the next minute? Their zone of optimal energy may be very small. A smaller zone of optimal energy may look like diverted attention, like Doug the dog in the movie *Up* who would be helping his owner on an important mission and then veer off, barking, "Squirrel!" Or a tiny zone of optimal energy may be quickly slipping into exhaustion, like my growing teenager in the morning.

We can enjoy the ebb and flow of our energy level automatically shifting with what the day and environment bring. We can also consciously and intentionally shift our energy level when ebbing and flowing is not going smoothly. Adjusting our energy level starts with being aware of our current energy level.

Recently, I realized I am much better at pouring the water into the coffee maker and putting ground coffee beans into the filter paper at night than I am in the morning. Seriously. In the morning, water spills and coffee grounds somehow end up on the counter, both annoying me and adding a clean-up job to my already busy morning. Making the coffee at night and turning on a timer is a better fit for me and my morning energy level.

A couple of months ago, I intensely felt the discrepancy between my energy level and what the day required. The day before, I had finished teaching a continuing education course to a group of therapists a couple of time zones away. I felt overjoyed and grateful for how well the course had gone. I was on cloud nine—so excited! I flew home and used that energy rush to reply to a lot of emails, and when I crawled into bed that night, I slept really hard. I woke up before my alarm went off, slightly disoriented by the angle of light and orientation of the room, having not been home for a couple of days, and then the exhaustion hit me like a ton of bricks. I opened my calendar app on my phone, and with only one eye partially open, I looked at my day. I was excited about teaching an online class and meeting with the leaders of our therapy center, Growing Healthy Seasons, but my energy level was really low. I knew the day's events needed my energy level to be higher. If my calendar for the day had been empty, this negative five energy level would have been a match, right? But it wasn't, and no amount of time management and prioritization would be the key to executing the day well. I needed to be alert and energetic, and for me, walking through my garden boosts my energy level, so that is what I did.

What can you do to adjust your energy level to match what is on your calendar for the day? Time management is part of a successful day, absolutely. You need to know whether each item on your To-Do list is urgent or important or both or neither.

But what if you don't even have the energy to make the To-Do list? And what if you have the beautiful list, all prioritized, but your energy level doesn't match any of the items on that list? Then the first thing on the calendar needs to be shifting your energy level, and that can be done through sensation. Just adding more caffeine is not sustainable for health, happiness, or optimization. If I were going to an amusement park or a rock concert, then maybe a bag of chocolate-covered espresso beans would work well for that day, but too many bags of espresso beans too often can create much bigger problems. The mismatch between actual energy level and desirable energy level is real-life me—and probably real-life you on some days! For your overall health and well-being, you can add sensations to your tools for shifting your energy level.

As you continue increasing your sensory awareness, let's look at some interesting and important research. Studies show if you have really high self-awareness and not enough self-regulation, that mismatch can lead to rumination, your brain rethinking about something over and over again when you want to be moving forward into action and regulation. Lots of self-awareness without regulation tools can also lead to increased anxiety and depression. Sensory regulation and self-awareness are so closely related, they're like superheroes that need each other in order to be their best, most powerful selves. We will work together to develop lots of regulation tools so you can be your best self and have the energy to live life to the fullest!

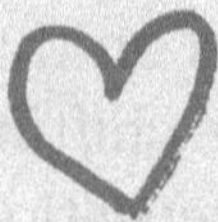

Energy Tracker:

Reflect: Fill out the "Energy Tracker" in your *Sensory Wellness Reflection Journal* or download the free resource from my website. Set an hourly alarm for every waking hour of your day for a whole week, rating your energy level each time the alarm goes off. What are the patterns of lower and higher energy levels throughout your days? What responsibilities can you reorganize to better match your energy level at different times of the day or week?

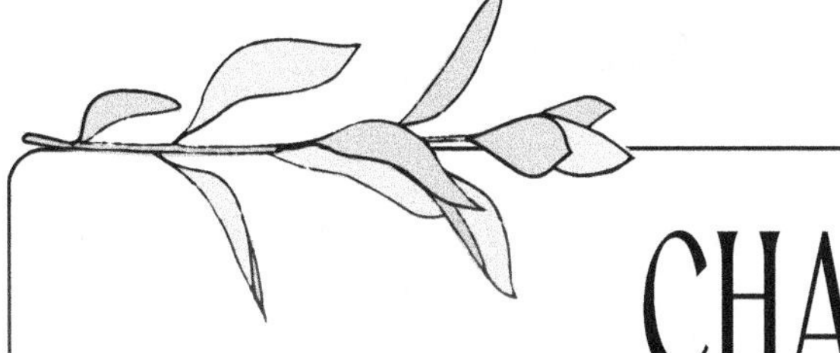

CHAPTER 12

The Power of Being Sensationally With: Deeper Connection

"We were together. I forget the rest."

- Walt Whitman -

Your regulation depends on the sensation around you in the form of other people too! You sense the sounds and sights of their breathing, fiddling, and movements. You detect their energy level and may pick up waves of their emotions. You are attuning unconsciously to those around you. *Attunement* is the ability to be aware of and respond to another person's emotions and needs, a pure tuning into other people's energy.

Studies, often on mother–young child pairs, show that physiologically, attunement can be observed and measured in breathing patterns, cortisol levels, heart rate variability, and facial expressions! In the brains of two people emotionally attuning, similar regions are activated in the *default mode network* (See appendix for more details on brain networks), the connections between the medial prefrontal cortex, amygdala, orbitofrontal cortex, and insula, among other areas of your brain. We form close relationships with people as we regularly attune to them and they attune to us. This pattern of perceiving how each other is doing allows us to feel connected to others and form emotional attachments. Too much tuning into others can be exhausting and codependent, and too little can be isolating and lonely. But just the right amount of attunement is the gateway to compassion and empathy. Mutually trusting interactions form deep connections, an indicator of overall health and well-being.

As an occupational therapist, one aspect I particularly love is being present with each family I work with. When the session starts, all elements of life outside the sensory play fade away, almost as if time stands still. I felt this in a session recently when I was playing with an eight-year-old boy, Skye, and his father.

I asked Skye, "What do you want to play today?"

As he ran over to the zip-line, his father chuckled because this was consistently his son's choice. We followed his lead, excited to see how the game would unfold as we created it. As the sensory therapist, I knew we were "officially" working on improving his core strength, motor coordination, and sensitivity to tactile information. The possibilities of how we would accomplish these goals together, through connected play, were endless! Skye started zooming past on the zip-line, and I sped over to him on a scooter board. Dad grabbed some weighted discs from the toy closet.

"What are those?" I asked.

"Donuts!" Dad shouted.

"I'll be the delivery man! Can I take your order?" Skye cheered.

And so, the game of *donut delivery man* was created! Being sensationally together made the game so fun, and people down the hall could hear all of us laughing for the next hour.

Chapter 12

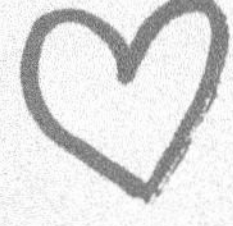

Increasing your awareness of attunement:

Reflect: Think of a time you reached out to a friend to process something or a time you felt connected to another. What did you feel in your body before connecting? What did you feel in your body after connecting?

The opposite of attunement has been studied at length, beginning with and most famously, Edward Tronick's "Still Face" experiment with babies (1978). In these studies, a mother is asked to interact with her baby and then stop, not responding or changing her facial expression at all. She does not look angry. Her facial expression is just flat, the inverse of attunement. The baby becomes distressed, bidding for attention and a response, with sounds and gestures. The baby's heart rate increases and breathing changes, and the baby's sympathetic nervous system activation increases. No longer feeling a sense of agency, the baby's stress increases.

The response of infants showing distress and attempting to re-engage the parent has been observed consistently across many diverse populations and cultures. This experiment has been replicated with older children, families of various cultures, children with different attachment patterns, parents with mental health challenges, children who were exposed to drugs *in utero*, children with Down syndrome, and autistic children, with many interesting insights. While neurodivergent children may have a variation in behavior indicating their expectations about social behavior, they also bid for a reaction from the adult.

"Every kid is one caring adult away from being a success story."

- Josh Shipp -

Sometimes we are less responsive to others or "still-face" people accidentally because we are disconnected from our bodies and the sensory world within and around us. We may be on a device and/or tuning the world out. When others still-face us, we can feel misunderstood, upset, frustrated, and stressed. There is harm caused when we still-face another person if we do not repair or reconnect afterward. The importance of validating emotions and being present with children is crucial because it sets a foundation for emotional regulation later in life. The dance of attunement and connection continues to be an essential component of sensory wellness for all ages.

But what if you don't feel good at attuning? Your ability to attune is partially related to your early attachment experiences with a parental figure. While early attachment is foundational to attunement, if attachment to your parents didn't go so well, you can still learn to attune and connect with others. Poor attachment then is not a death sentence for good attachment now. One way to get better at attuning is to become more in tune with your own emotions.

And guess what emotions are? Emotions are your brain and body making sense of sensation in the present with the lens of past experiences! Starting with increased awareness of both your interoceptive and exteroceptive sensation, you can increase your perception of feelings and your emotional vocabulary. Emotions are consultants, giving you information. They don't get to be in charge all the time.

Chapter 12

Attunement is powerful: starting with sensation and growing into emotion. Be sensationally with someone today!

All of us have people in our circles of connection, concentric rings that represent the depth of relationship and interaction we have with others. The outer circle is for people who are more like acquaintances or people you don't know very well but are in your life regularly. As you move closer to the center, the depth of relationship and connection increases. The inner circle is the place for those you feel the safest being around. People who you love, and they love you, not despite your vulnerability and imperfections, but because of them. They will point out when you are doing something that is not in line with your core values. Ideally, the people in your innermost circle of connection are people who care enough about you to be honest with you, rather than telling you what you want to hear. They are not people who just blindly agree with you no matter what. When you mess up, they will help you make things right. That inner circle is small on purpose: it is reserved for those who have earned the right to an opinion on your life.

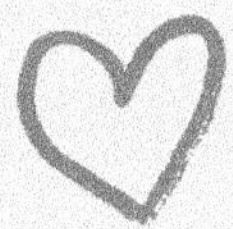

Circles of connection: increasing your awareness

Do: In your *Sensory Wellness Reflection Journal* or on the "Circles of Connection" resource on my website, write down the names of the people you know in the connection circles based on the closeness of your relationship. Whom do you choose to be in your inner circle of connection and attunement?

Reflect: Do you find yourself listening to criticism from people who aren't in your inner circle?

"When we define ourselves by what everyone thinks, it's hard to be brave. When we stop caring about what anyone thinks, we're too armored for authentic connection."

- Brené Brown -

Be intentional about entrusting the best people to influence and guide you. Some people are worthy, absolutely. Some are not. You get to choose your inner circle. Who are you with when you are the best version of yourself? Your answer will be different for each season of life.

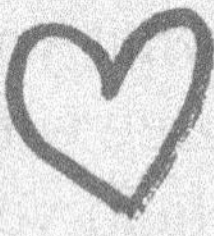

Circles of connection: changing with intention

Reflect:

- ✦ Who has impacted your regulation recently? Are they in your inner circle?
- ✦ Whom have you attuned to? Did they impact your energy level?
- ✦ After thinking about whom you want in your inner circle, is there anyone you want to kick out? Anyone you would like to move out to a different circle?

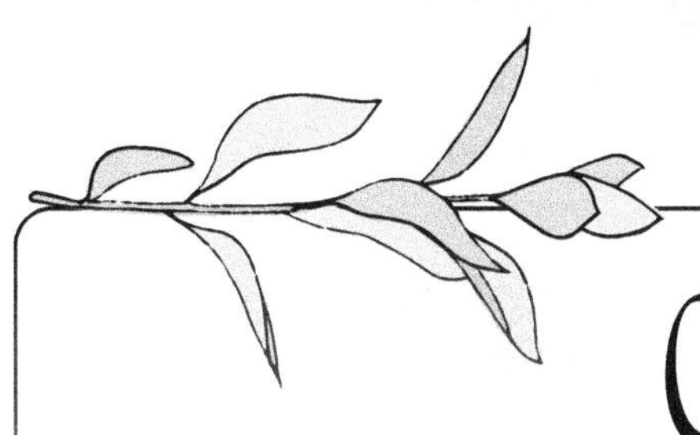

CHAPTER 13

Sensory Strategies for Thriving

"Life is not about waiting for the storm to pass,
it is about learning to dance in the rain."

- Vivian Greene -

Te power of sensation: sensing is living. Every cell in your body senses in different ways. Just take a moment to breathe in the reality of that! You are so alive! Even when you are so tired you don't feel like you can move, your body is sensing within yourself and outside of yourself. The key to sensory wellness is intentional sensory changes based on what your sensory awareness is telling you. Reinhold Niebuhr's serenity prayer with some sensory flair says it so well:

God, grant me the serenity
to accept the sensation I cannot change;
courage to change the sensations I can;
and wisdom to know the difference.

When choosing sensory strategies to thrive and help you be the best you, consider these four questions:

- Do I like or dislike this sensation?
- Do I want more or less of this sensation?

- Does this sensation shift my energy level?
- If this sensation shifts my energy level, how?

Bonus! The questions of, "Do I like it?" and, "Do I want more or less of this sensation?" are both connected to internal sensation processing (interoception). So as you explore these sensory strategies, you are supporting your interoceptive awareness and continuing to develop an intentional partnership with your body. Start up a conversation with your body as you try out sensory tools and listen deeply.

Let's warm up to the idea of using sensation as a tool with a sensation so simple and constant we may overlook it: Light! How can I change the lighting to help me do what is next on my schedule?

It's been a long week. So many responsibilities on the home front, family activities, and work responsibilities. I'm so close to being done for the day, but then I remember, I have one more thing to do: review paperwork for my team. I was supposed to get it done all week, and I can't put it off another day, nor do I want it hanging over my head all weekend. So I look around the room. It is getting dark outside, and the fluorescent light in this room, with its rapid flickering, has been bothering me all day. Now it is unbearable. Let's think through the questions from above:

- Do I like or dislike this sensation? *I do not like this fluorescent light.*
- Do I want more or less of this sensation? *I want less of it, right now.*
- Does this sensation shift my energy level? Yes! *The fluorescent light is shifting my sensory arousal level, and not in a helpful way!*

- ✦ If this sensation shifts my energy level, how? *Stealing the little bit of energy I have, the light is sucking all of my energy when I try to block it out.*

I look around the room and see my diffuser that has a setting that imitates a candle. Yes, still a variable visual input. But so different! I turn it on and start reviewing the paperwork—so much better!

A tool is a tool for right now if it doesn't bother those around me and works here in this place.

As we go through the sensory systems and explore sensory options that you may want to add to the sensory supportive lifestyle you are creating, remember that some tools will not match *where* you are at the moment or may not work well with *who* you are around. For instance, my pillow that plays music through vibration and helps me sleep at night won't be a good option to bring to a tricky meeting at a school, even though it does calm me down. Or blasting my favorite music in the car? Yes, it wakes me up and gets me ready for my day, but it also frustrates my kids. Can you imagine the exasperated, "Mom!" and the exaggerated eye roll?

Responses from my clients:

"*I've adjusted the lighting for a long time! Now I know why!*"

So fun! As you explore these tools, you may find things you have always done a certain way make so much more sense now. Fantastic! Understanding the *why* will help you prioritize the strategy when things get busy or hard. Have a weighted blanket? A favorite hairbrush? A preference for matched scented shampoo and conditioners? Use it!

"*I don't have time for this. I am already too busy taking care of my family and people at work.*"

You don't have time *not* to prioritize this. You need to take care of yourself so you can take care of others. I get it. I had a realization when my kids were young, and we were flying to Colorado on a work trip. The flight attendants did their regular spiel. I heard them say, "In the event of a sudden loss of pressure in the cabin, oxygen masks will drop from the overhead compartments. Parents of young children, put your own oxygen mask on first." Then they were required to walk down the aisle, confirming understanding of this concept with every parent. I nodded and realized the application of this instruction.

I was *not* doing this in life. Instead of putting my oxygen mask on first, I was trying to blow out fires with my own lung capacity day in and day out as the cabin pressure of my life took a nose dive.

I remember feeling so confused about the concept of a Sabbath for a mom of young children. Take a break? So, no one eats? The dishes stack up? Kids run around in chaos, fighting? Toys spread everywhere? My heart rate went up at the thought of what the day after Sabbath would look like. Put on my oxygen mask first? Take care of myself? I couldn't remember the last time I had eaten food that was still warm.

Looking back with love and empathy, I realize that I took a lot on that wasn't mine to carry. I had developed some unhealthy life patterns of people-pleasing and codependency that were not doing me any favors. So, as I write this, I get it, and, yes, I'm telling you these tools are for you—the working professional, parent, grandparent, caregiver, or teacher—so you can keep caring, you can keep breathing.

Chapter 13

These sensory tools will help you grow and bloom and flourish! By using sensory tools, you'll create the foundation to then implement and put into practice all the training and skills in prioritization, time management, and efficiency you have learned throughout your life. Power is in the sensory tools unlocking your abilities. Let's start bridging the gap between your ideal sensory world and your reality. Let's close the distance between your energy needs and your current energy level.

"*I feel lost. Are there any common patterns or clues to start with?*"

Many, but not all, people feel increased energy and alertness with intermittent, variable sensation. Unpredictable and more intense input will also increase most people's energy level, getting more of their brain's attention. And the opposite pattern is often true as well: predictable, steady, controllable, and less intense input will likely decrease people's alertness level and be more calming. But I have observed and heard of so many exceptions. We are all so different, in such a beautiful way. One unpredictable sound might throw my stress response into a quick spike of activation. Whereas for someone else, it might take one hundred unpredictable sounds to barely make their stress response jump up a little. So, try the tools and strategies with an open mind. There are no, "I should feel," no wrong answers, just your most authentic and true perception of your experience.

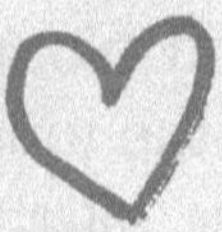

One challenging part of my life:

Reflect: To put this into practice in your life and prevent it from just being a fun series of random sensory activities and ideas, think about a hard thing you do in life regularly right now. Is it interacting with a certain person? Is it the bedtime routine? Waking up in the morning? Take a moment to record your challenge in your *Sensory Wellness Reflection Journal.* We are going to apply each of these sets of tools to that situation or task to help the concepts root in your brain.

"There is a voice that doesn't use words. Listen."

~ Rumi ~

Visual Tools

Try these ideas for changing the visual sensation around you:

- ✦ Hang something on the wall that makes you smile.
- ✦ Change the lighting.
- ✦ Look at an oil-and-water bottle.
- ✦ Clear the counters.
- ✦ Shift the direction your desk faces.
- ✦ Put up fluorescent light covers.
- ✦ Change the color theme—accents, rugs, art.

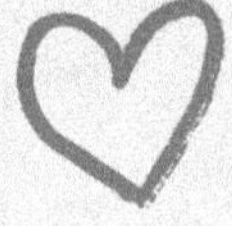

Do: Try each of these or other visual sensation activities and check in with your body. Do I like or dislike this sensation? Do I want more or less of this sensation? Again, no wrong answer here. Each person is different in the way sensation impacts them.

My sister has a bookshelf in her dining room. Everyone saw the bookshelf every day. One day, she and her daughter moved the books around to be organized by color, and everyone in the family noticed and loved the new look. It shifted the energy and interactions around the dinner table. These sensory environment changes don't fix huge problems, but they do make a difference in daily life.

Here are some ideas to help you notice how visual sensation can shift your energy:

- Watch a fire in a fireplace.
- Watch a sunrise or sunset.
- Work with fluorescent lighting on.
- Look at a lava lamp.
- Gaze at an oil-and-water scene.

Record what you notice in your *Sensory Wellness Reflection Journal* or the "Sensory Tools Checklist" from the resources section of my website. How do these sensations increase or decrease your energy level? Do you feel more alert? Or do you feel calmer and more relaxed? Has your breathing and/or heart rate slowed down? Some sensory tools might not change your energy level at all and others may both increase and decrease your energy level depending on the situation.

Reflect:

- What colors support you in feeling more alert and energized?
- What colors help you feel calmer and more relaxed?

Back to that challenge in life right now you thought of earlier:

When I was a high jumper in college, I used to visualize myself jumping over the bar and not knocking it over. Professional athletes do this visualization as part of their training. They lean into the crucial moment, and instead of disconnecting from their bodies, they feel all the senses as much as possible. Now, it is your turn. Let's light up all those networks in your brain and make the challenge you thought of earlier better. Visualize the vision component of the challenge and then visualize it getting less hard. What can you shift visually to make this not as bad?

- What does it look like?
- What is one thing you can shift sight-wise to make your challenge more pleasant?

Auditory Tools

Try these ideas for changing the auditory sensation around you:

- Turn on background music.
- Put on noise-canceling headphones.
- Use a sound machine.
- Soundproof your space.
- Turn off phone and computer notifications.

Do: Try each of these or other auditory sensation activities and check in with your body. Do I like or dislike this sensation? Do I want more or less of this sensation? All answers are good: be sensationally you!

Chapter 13

The first time I wore noise-canceling headphones on a plane, I felt like I was at the spa! Okay, maybe not quite, but close! I was floored by how lovely the experience was! My sister had let me borrow her high-quality noise-canceling headphones for a cross-country flight. I was traveling for work and had so much to get done on the plane ride: review reports, edit a paper, enhance a presentation. On most flights, I perceive the energy of those around me and sincerely enjoy meeting new people, learning about their journey. But for this trip, I needed to be on my top get-it-done game, and those noise-canceling headphones were effective! What a gift!

Do you notice sound bouncing around your workspace, magnifying the noise with extra reverberations? Do those mini echoes help you thrive, or sound like nails on a chalkboard? There are so many types of soundproofing if you want to turn down the extra noise, including corner triangles, fabric panels, heavy-duty construction materials, and cute soundproofing pictures. Explore some options if you feel that would be helpful!

Here are some ideas to help you notice how auditory sensation can shift your energy:

- ✦ Work in a quiet room.
- ✦ Work in a noisy room.
- ✦ Sing or talk to yourself.
- ✦ Listen to classical music.
- ✦ Awaken to an unusual noise.

Record what you notice in your *Sensory Wellness Reflection Journal* or the “Sensory Tools Checklist” from the resources section of my website. How do these sensations increase or decrease your energy level? Some might not change your energy level at all and others may both increase and decrease your energy level depending on the situation.

Even if you need to wait a little while to reflect on how these auditory tools shift your energy, do one thing right now. Open up the settings on your phone or computer, and go to Notifications. Check your apps and ask yourself, are these the settings for notifications I want? Are vibration or sound alarms going off that I don't want to interrupt my day? Which of your contacts do you want to be able to break through your focus mode? Do alerts about what friends and family are posting on social media help you maintain a motivated and alert energy level throughout the day, or are the alerts draining? When your phone buzzes, your stress response increases a little. Remember, the stress response is not a good or bad thing inherently. You get to decide whether the activation serves you and helps you be who you want to be and do what you want to do.

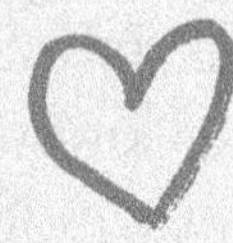

Reflect:

- ✦ What songs support you in feeling more alert and energized?
- ✦ What songs help you feel calmer and more relaxed?

Back to your challenge:

- ✦ What does it sound like?
- ✦ What is one thing you can shift sound-wise to make your challenge more pleasant?

Tactile Tools

Try these ideas for changing your tactile sensation:

- ✦ Hold a fidget.
- ✦ Place a soft blanket or pillow on your lap.
- ✦ Apply your favorite lotion.
- ✦ Wear comfortable clothes.

- ✦ Invite a pet to sit on you or lean against you.
- ✦ Sit on a comfy chair or sofa.
- ✦ Change your keyboard or add a keyboard cover.
- ✦ Choose jewelry based on sensation.
- ✦ Put a hair tie or rubber band on your wrist.

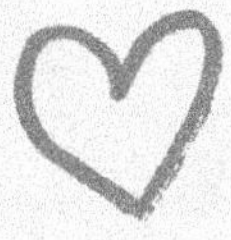

Do: Try each of these or other tactile sensation activities and check in with your body. Do I like or dislike this sensation? Do I want more or less of this sensation?

I'm not sure if it was the years of working only from home or being in my forties or some combination, but my tolerance for uncomfortable clothes has disappeared. Cute? Yes. Uncomfortable? No tight waistbands? Tight legs? Actually, tight most things? No thank you. I'm not wearing it. It started with the business-on-top-and-pajamas-on-the-bottom style of the pandemic years and just expanded from there. Luckily, soft fabrics and loose waist options abound.

Whether considering the options for shoes, sandals, and slippers or haircuts, the power comes from thinking about how the tactile sensation of each option will help you be your best self or hinder you. You get to choose, on purpose.

Here are some ideas to help you notice how tactile sensation can shift your energy:

- ✦ Take a cool shower.
- ✦ Enjoy a hot bath.
- ✦ Receive a massage.
- ✦ Drum fingers or pencil.
- ✦ Gently touch skin or clothes.

Record what you notice in your *Sensory Wellness Reflection Journal* or the "Sensory Tools Checklist" from the resources section of my website. How do these sensations increase or decrease your energy level? Some might not change your energy level at all and others may both increase and decrease your energy level depending on the situation.

Reflect:

- ✦ What types of clothing help you feel more alert and energized?
- ✦ What types of clothing help you feel calmer and more relaxed?

Back to your challenge:

- ✦ What does it feel like (touch-wise)?
- ✦ What is one thing you can shift touch-wise to make your challenge more pleasant?

Olfactory Tools

Try these ideas for changing the olfactory sensation around you:

- ✦ Use different shampoo and conditioner.
- ✦ Try new hair products.
- ✦ Diffuse essential oils.
- ✦ Light a scented candle or use a candle warming plate.
- ✦ Burn incense.
- ✦ Grow scented plants around (inside and/or outside).
- ✦ Arrange a bouquet of flowers.
- ✦ Drink coffee or tea.

When I think about becoming clear on what sensation you can and cannot control, the first thing I think about is laundry detergent. I borrowed a sweatshirt from a good friend a couple years ago and loved the way it smelled. The scent seemed to say, "I'm amazing, and I have my life together. I'm a great mom and an awesome professional, and I've got the home front dialed in! I might even iron clothing sometimes!" All that with a scent! And then it occurred to me: I could ask her about the laundry detergent brand and scent and use it too. Then the smell of my clothes could be encouraging to me. This is something I have agency about—I get to choose.

Do: Try each of these or other olfactory sensation activities and check in with your body. Do I like or dislike this sensation? Do I want more or less of this sensation?

Here are some ideas to help you notice how olfactory sensation can shift your energy:

- Take a big whiff of garlic cooking.
- Add lavender oil to your lip gloss.
- Boil cinnamon in water.
- Chew peppermint gum.
- Place an air freshener in your car.

Record what you notice in your *Sensory Wellness Reflection Journal* or the "Sensory Tools Checklist" from the resources section of my website. How do these sensations increase or decrease your energy level? Some might not change your energy level at all and others may both increase and decrease your energy level depending on the situation.

Reflect:

- ✦ What scents support you feeling more alert and energized?
- ✦ What scents help you feel calmer and more relaxed?

Back to your challenge:

- ✦ Does it have a smell? If so, what does it smell like?
- ✦ What is one thing you can shift smell-wise to make your challenge more pleasant?

Gustatory Tools

Try eating and drinking these foods for changing your taste sensations:

- ✦ Spicy food
- ✦ Sweet treats
- ✦ Sour food
- ✦ Mint, cucumber, lemon in your water
- ✦ Thicker liquids (smoothie-ish) with a straw

Over the years, I have tended to think of what I am going to eat based on what is deemed "healthy" by the current theories. More veggies, more fruit, more coconut oil, more avocados, no eggs, but wait! Yes, eggs! Or I have gravitated toward what I'm craving: dark chocolate and coffee.

Yes, flourless chocolate cake is amazing, but like my friend says, "Is it an everyday food or a sometimes food?" Not to mention the unhelpful crash that often comes after too much. A different approach from relying on sugar and caffeine, which can have lasting negative side effects, can also be helpful in increasing your focus and energy. Let's talk about a few.

One healthier way to increase alertness is to add or decrease spice or add something sour to a snack. You can also purposely make your smoothie a bit thicker and drink it through a small straw. Freeze grapes and eat them after they have thawed the tiniest bit. The flavors combined with the increased proprioceptive input of your jaw muscles working hard will support your active efforts to adjust your energy level and overall regulation. So, enjoy some taste tools, shifting some of your meal choices and elements to help you be where you need to be with your energy level.

Do: Try each of these or other gustatory sensation activities and check in with your body. Do I like or dislike this sensation? Do I want more or less of this sensation? Remember no wrong answers and no "I should" here.

Here are some ideas to help you notice how taste sensations can shift your energy:

- Crunch ice pieces.
- Eat a pickle.
- Eat spicy food.
- Drink coffee or tea.
- Crunch on something salty like nuts, pretzels. or chips.

Record what you notice in your *Sensory Wellness Reflection Journal* or the "Sensory Tools Checklist" from the resources section of my website. How do these sensations increase or decrease your energy level? Some might not change your energy level at all and others may both increase and decrease your energy level depending on the situation.

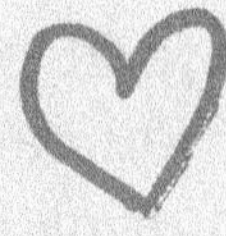

Reflect:

- What tastes support you in feeling more alert and energized?
- What tastes help you feel calmer and more relaxed?

Back to your challenge:

- Does it have a taste? If so, what is the taste of it?
- What is one thing you can shift taste-wise to make your challenge more pleasant?

Proprioceptive (Muscles and Joints) Tools

Remember the proprioceptive receptors: muscle fibers contracting and relaxing, joints pushing together and pulling apart, receptors deep in your skin. Crucial for your overall well-being, proprioceptive input initiates the cascade of happy neurotransmitters in your brain. Research shows that proprioceptive input can impact your regulation and sensory processing for multiple hours.

Try these ideas to change your proprioceptive sensation:

- Hand strengthener: Use a tool with springs to resist your muscles' contracting to make a fist or squeeze a tennis ball.
- Tongue pushups: Push your tongue to the top of your mouth and count to five. Then relax your mouth muscles. Repeat as preferred.
- Toe Squeezes: Curl your toes up under your feet and count to five. Then relax your foot and calf muscles. Repeat as preferred.
- Hairline massage: Place your fingers along your hairline and massage the skin.

- Breathing techniques: There are so many choices! The simplest one I love is focusing on breathing out longer than you breathe in.
- Weighted blanket or lap animal (stuffed toy or real).
- Therapy ball to sit or lie on.
- Yoga break cards.
- Hanging bar in doorway: Put a pull-up bar in a doorway. Instead of (or in addition to) doing pull-ups, try hanging on the bar.
- Handheld massager: Move device slowly and gently over a muscle group, avoiding putting direct pressure on bones and joints.
- Resistance bands: Place on forearms and pull your hands away from each other and then slowly bring them back together. Or put the band above your knees and pull your legs apart.

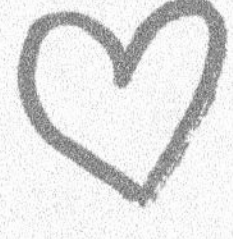

Do: Try each of these or other proprioceptive sensation activities and check in with your body. Do I like or dislike this sensation? Do I want more or less of this sensation?

Here are some ideas to help you notice how proprioceptive sensation can shift your energy:

- Lift weights or do isometric exercises.
- Stretch.
- Tap toes or heels while sitting.
- Shift your body while sitting
- Roll your head slowly from side to side

Record what you notice in your *Sensory Wellness Reflection Journal* or the "Sensory Tools Checklist" from the resources section of my website. How do these sensations increase or decrease your energy level? Some might not change your energy level at all and others may both increase and decrease your energy level depending on the situation.

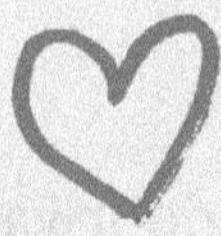

Reflect:

- ✦ What activities using your muscles and joints support you in feeling more alert and energized?
- ✦ What activities using your muscles and joints help you feel calmer and more relaxed?

Back to your challenge:

- ✦ What are your muscles doing during the challenge?
- ✦ What is one thing you can shift, body position and muscle contraction-wise, to make your challenge more pleasant?

Vestibular (Movement and Balance) Tools

Remember, vestibular receptors are in your inner ear and detect movement changes, supporting balance and posture in addition to cognitive function and mood, even decreasing anxiety in some studies. Brief movement input can shift your brain activation and regulation for minutes and even hours! You can start connecting with your vestibular system by sitting on the ground for a couple minutes each day.

Try these ideas for ways to change your vestibular input:

- ✦ Spin in an office chair.
- ✦ Hang a reminder/happy picture on the ceiling and look up at it from time to time.
- ✦ Invert yourself (fancy table or lying over the edge of your bed with your head close to the floor).
- ✦ Jog or walk.

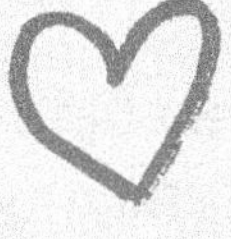

Do: Try each of these or other vestibular sensation activities and check in with your body. Do I like or dislike this sensation? Do I want more or less of this sensation?

Here are some ideas to help you notice how vestibular sensation can shift your energy:

- ✦ Rock in a rocking chair.
- ✦ Lean chair back on two legs.
- ✦ Ride a bike.
- ✦ Swing (on a hammock, tree swing, playground swing).
- ✦ Put your head between your knees.

Record what you notice in your *Sensory Wellness Reflection Journal* or the "Sensory Tools Checklist" from the resources section of my website. How do these sensations increase or decrease your energy level? Some might not change your energy level at all and others may both increase and decrease your energy level depending on the situation.

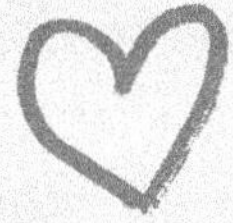

Reflect:

- ✦ What movement activities help you feel more alert and energized?
- ✦ What movement activities help you feel calmer and more relaxed?

Back to your challenge:

- ✦ What movement does it include?
- ✦ What is one thing you can shift movement-wise to make your challenge more pleasant?

Sensory Threshold: The minimal intensity of a sensory input needed for a person to detect the sensation, notice a change in the level of input, or become overwhelmed by the sensation.

Sensory Thresholds

Our bodies and brains are wired to bring attention to *sensory thresholds*. We notice when an element of our environment shifts from part of the noise of life (an air conditioner turning on and off or the buzz of the refrigerator working) to potentially mission critical (the front door opening). This sensory threshold helps us save our energy for what we need to pay attention to.

For some people, their sensory threshold may be at a problematically low level: their brain is sending out warning messages with every little sensation. Too low of a threshold ends up disrupting everyday life: a nice meal at a restaurant feels like a warzone of sensation bombarding a person's body. The tag in the shirt feels like a razor blade. Life is screaming at the person.

Too high of a sensory threshold can also be problematic! It could be embarrassing if your clothes were twisted funny and your skin didn't tell you to adjust. Delayed or decreased registering sensation can be dangerous as well! You go to move a pan on the stove, and your skin doesn't tell you the pan is too hot? You get burned! You start crossing the street and you don't register the car coming around the corner? You almost get hit! If a person has too high of a threshold for sensation, they don't perceive sensation until the last moment and maybe not at all.

And then there is another sensory threshold when our bodies and brains say, "Too much!" We are also wired to respond to a level of sensation is overwhelming: not helpful, intolerable, and definitely not enjoyable. We cover our ears when there is a loud car alarm going off. We open the windows when the trash didn't get taken out and now the house smells awful.

High and low sensory thresholds can be related to genetics, a neurodevelopmental difference, a traumatic event, among other factors. While each person's sensory thresholds have a different baseline and can vary day to day, we all have these sensory thresholds. Amazingly, your sensory threshold for one type of sensation can be shifted intentionally using other sensations.

A teenaged girl, Sam, came to see me because the "ick" factor of life was so frustrating for her. While Sam's sensitivity to tactile input had been making many aspects of life hard for a long time, the last straw that made her want to shift her sensory processing was that now this low sensory threshold was messing up her social life. Sam wanted to tolerate the jeans all her friends were wearing, but they hurt her skin too much. She wanted to eat the food her friends were eating at the local hangout spots, but she couldn't touch a French fry, much less eat one! So, we worked together on shifting her threshold, using her proprioceptive, vestibular and olfactory senses.

Over the course of a couple months, Sam learned about her sensory thresholds and we made a plan together. Sam climbed up layers of Lycra hammocks, contracting her muscles to stabilize herself. She set personal records balancing on a large blow-up pillow bigger than a king-sized bed. She rocked on a swing, slow and steady, while brainstorming holiday gifts for her friends. And we worked together to make salt scrubs with different calming scents. The textures of the salt scrub ingredients were hard at first. Over time, Sam's threshold for tactile input increased and she started feeling more at ease hanging out with her friends. She found some jeans that didn't hurt her skin and fit the style she was going for.

Thresholds can also change temporarily depending on what is going on around you. Let's imagine that you just enjoyed a quiet retreat week, the loudest sounds you heard were the birds greeting the sun and the waves crashing on the shore. You drive home reflecting on your week and planning the next couple days of meals and schedules. When you pull in the driveway, familiar sounds greet you: the buzz of a busy household full of kids laughing, crying, fighting, and playing. What was a basic, regular level of sounds that your body was used to, now feels like the clanging of pots and pans. You notice your eyes wincing and your shoulders tightening. Your sensory threshold for overwhelm shifted over the week away. Over time, your auditory system will adjust back, shifting the level of sensation that feels like too much. These threshold changes are normal. We can notice them, listen in, and adjust.

Sensory tools are powerful in shifting the way you experience life: both in changing thresholds and sensation in a moment in time! You have the agency to change more than you ever consciously thought about. So now that you have a better sense of what sensory tools support the energy level you need to do what you want to do, how do you incorporate these into your daily life for a sensationally supportive lifestyle? Turning what you explored in this chapter into healthy life habits and routines will take a little time but is worth it! Let's cultivate this sensational life more together.

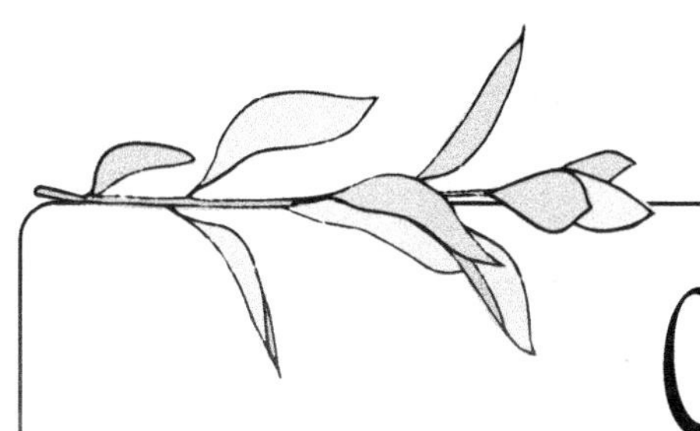

CHAPTER 14

Cultivating Sensory Wellness: The Pillars of Health

"When you take the time to replenish your spirit, it allows you to serve others from overflow. You cannot serve from an empty vessel."

- Eleanor Brown -

How do you make sure you are well enough to help others in your job and in your home? Sensory wellness is so much more than self-love or self-care. We are not talking about just buying a new toothbrush or going to yoga. Sensory wellness is thriving so you can live out your purpose, being the best you you can be. Originally developed by the American College of Lifestyle Medicine and adapted for sensory wellness, the multi-sensory pillars of health will help you thrive. As we dig deep into some practical components of health, you can apply these ideas to your journey as it makes sense to do so and considering any medical conditions you are working through currently. Apply this information individually and in the context of your medication for anxiety, chemotherapy, nutrition plan for an autoimmune disorder, or other medical needs. These basic concepts of health can be incorporated into your wellness plan with the support of medical and mental health professionals when needed. The pillars of health may be your first clue that something in your body or brain needs help along your health journey. If you are sensing red flags, now is the time to call a medical professional to get some tests, possibly lab work to look into the health of your blood, kidneys, thyroid, etc. As you increase your internal and external sensory awareness, your senses will help guide you to the answers you need to flourish!

I felt the power of sensation in guiding myself to health a couple of years ago. I have always loved having a full plate of activities and roles, with a lot going on. I felt energized by navigating a tricky schedule and have done my best work when I have a lot to do. However, as I tuned into my sensory cues, I began to notice my energy level was often very low, and I was dysregulated much of the time. I started to take more and more events off my schedule and was still not feeling rested. My body was telling me something was going on, so I got some lab work done as a first step. Sure enough, my B-12, zinc, and iron were very low and my selenium was very high (didn't realize my affinity for Brazil nuts could be dangerous).

Whether you take a Western, Eastern, holistic, specialist, naturopathic, or other approach, listen to your body if it is telling you something is not quite right and reach out for help.

The pillars of health are made up of different combinations of sensation. Most people would say, "I want to be healthy," but the idea of making changes in your life to be healthier can be overwhelming. What do you prioritize? Which one of the over 177.6 million podcasts full of ideas do you listen to first? What if two podcasts offer contradictory suggestions? In all seasons of life, I want to flourish like the tree Jeremiah describes in the Bible: a tree planted by the water that sends roots by the stream, not fearing when heat comes, leaves always green, not worrying in a year of drought, never failing to bear fruit. So how do we get there? Let's stick to the basics and stay rooted in sensory integration, exploring the pillars of health together and continuing the journey of sensory wellness!

The Pillars of Health

Sleep

Nutrition

Movement

Connection

Contemplative Practice

Play & Leisure

Sleep

"By helping us keep the world in perspective, sleep gives us a chance to refocus on the essence of who we are. And in that place of connection, it is easier for the fears and concerns of the world to drop away."

- Arianna Huffington -

Sleep makes all the other pillars of health stronger, so we are going to start here. While you can't force your body to go to sleep (trying just makes it worse for me), you can break down the components of healthy sleeping and then make adjustments in the sensory areas you need to in order to support getting the best sleep you can.

Your sleep health can be measured by your QQRT (quantity, quality, regularity, timing): the combination of the quantity of sleep you are getting, the quality of the sleep, the regularity, and the timing of your sleep compared to your natural chronotype (the time when you naturally feel most alert and productive during the day and the time when you prefer to sleep). For quantity, most adults need seven to nine hours of sleep per night. The quality of your sleep is related to staying asleep as much as possible and your sleep cycles. While many people wake up briefly and then drift back into sleep cycles a couple times a night, frequent and prolonged awakenings, can decrease the quality of your sleep. If you wake up twenty times a night, your quality of sleep score will be low even if you sleep for twelve hours. It is best to go to sleep and wake up at consistent times every day. A high regularity score would be a regular time plus or minus thirty minutes. So if I'm often setting my alarm for six, I will have a higher regularity score if I wake up between 5:30 and 6:30 a.m. every day. Research has shown that sleeping in to catch-up on sleep, even one or two days per week, is not supportive of the best sleep health. A good score on the timing of your sleep is if your sleep schedule matches your circadian rhythm or natural chronotype. You can learn about if you tend to be more of a morning person or an evening person by taking the Morningness-Eveningness Questionnaire (MEQ) by James Horne Olov Östberg that is free online (1976). The basic idea of your natural chronotype is that if you got to wave a magic wand and your schedule was not dictated by your job, your partner, your kids, or your pets, when would you prefer to sleep?

What is the impact of quality sleep on your overall health and wellness? Research shows, good sleep cleans your brain and heals your heart and blood vessels. Sleep helps you have a healthy balance of the hormones that tell you if you are full or hungry: you will feel hungrier if you are tired! Sleep supports the regulation of your blood glucose (sugar) level and boosts your immune system functioning. Additionally, good sleep supports puberty and fertility. Quality sleep even decreases your risk of heart disease, high blood pressure, obesity, and stroke! And then there is the neuroscience side of it! Sleep supports our ability to think clearly, file memories, regulate emotions, and focus. It also increases neuroplasticity. Someone who is sleep-deprived responds to low-level stressors similar to how a well-rested person responds to a high-level stressor!

***Neuroplasticity*:** The brain's remarkable ability to reorganize neural connections (think map of roads) by forming new connections throughout life, adapting to new experiences, learning new skills, recovering from injury, and adjusting to changing circumstances.

Multi-Sensory Sleep Health Strategies

- ✦ Get sunlight exposure early in the day.
- ✦ Reduce blue light exposure from screens at night.
- ✦ Have a calming and consistent bedtime routine.
- ✦ Exercise (but not too much or too late).
- ✦ Intentionally eat food to nourish your brain and body (too little fat or carbohydrates can impair sleep).
- ✦ Use calming breathing techniques.
- ✦ Keep the bedroom completely dark (blackout curtains).
- ✦ Maintain a cool to cold bedroom temperature.
- ✦ Listen to white noise or relaxing music.
- ✦ Avoid sleep-interrupting foods and drinks, like chocolate, coffee, and alcohol, for 4 hours before bedtime

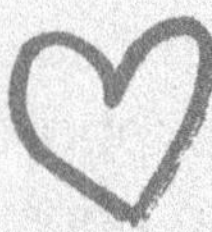

Sleep Reflections:

- ✦ What is your sleep like currently?
- ✦ What feelings and sensations do you notice when you get your best sleep?
- ✦ What shifts can you make to your sensory environment to support improving your sleep?
- ✦ Does your sleep routine recharge you enough?

Nutrition

"Let food be thy medicine and medicine be thy food."
- Hippocrates -

The starting point for the nutrition pillar of health is choosing foods to eat to nourish your soul, body, and mind. Eat so you can do what you love. Instead of focusing on foods you need to limit or eliminate, focus on what foods you want to eat more of and on hydrating in order to be your best self. You can choose foods to help you sleep better, adjust your hormones, give you an extra boost of energy, increase your mental clarity, or comfort you. Eat intentionally and strategically to do what you love.

This pillar of health is not meant to tell you exactly what food you should eat. I don't like "shoulds," and I try to stay away from them when possible. Additionally, your ideal diet is deeply individual, based on your genetics, culture, allergies, way of processing food, overall wellness, and health challenges. So if you are feeling the need to make a big shift, decide on a ketogenic; gluten-free, casein-free (GFCF); vegan; vegetarian; pescatarian; Fermentable, Oligosaccharides, Disaccharides, Monosaccharides and Polyols (FODMAP); or other diet with a registered dietitian or other qualified healthcare professional. You may find getting blood work done and providing a stool sample helpful as a baseline on your wellness journey.

One thing is clear across all people: we need to eat foods that have nutrients, real food. We also need to make sure our nutritional needs are being met. Our bodies need carbohydrates, proteins, fats, vitamins, minerals, and water. These nutrients keep our bodies healthy, sustaining body functions, providing energy, building and repairing tissues, and regulating our bodily processes. We know fresh food has the most nutrients. If you eat an apple off the tree, you get more nutrients than if that apple was picked six months ago. The longer a food takes to get to your table, the fewer nutrients it contains. Making sure to eat a variety of nutrients regularly reduces your risk of diabetes, heart disease, and stroke. Nutrients improve your immune system functioning, helping you fight off or recover from a flu or cold. Nutrients also improve your mood and support your mental health, decreasing anxiety and depression.

The research is also conclusive that all people benefit from avoiding certain things. Smoking, vaping, alcohol, and recreational drugs hurt your body and brain. Foods with pesticides, antibiotics, added growth hormones, preservatives, artificial ingredients, chemicals, synthetic food dyes, and plastics not only cause physiological damage, but also decrease focus, increase hyper-sensitivity, and have long-term impacts.

With the general goal of eating food with nutritional value and avoiding the conclusively harmful options, how do you choose what food to eat? Most of the middle of grocery stores is processed and contains fewer nutrients. Mostly shop the border of the store and go to farmers markets or farms when possible. If you cannot pronounce an ingredient on the food label, it is wise to limit or avoid that food.

In an effort to do what is important to you, eat to fuel yourself. Have an ongoing conversation between you and your body about the specific foods you decide to eat for a meal or snack:

- ✦ How do I feel when I am eating this food?
- ✦ How much of this food do I eat before I feel full?
- ✦ How do I feel after I eat this food?
- ✦ How much energy do I have after I eat this? For how long?
- ✦ How long does it take before I feel hungry again?

Recent research has illuminated the connection between your *microbiome* and wellness. The microbiome is a community of trillions of microorganisms living in your gut, on your skin, surrounding your internal organs, and in your vaginal and nasal mucous membranes. Healthy microorganisms, including good bacteria, fungi, viruses, and other microbes, support digestion, nutrient absorption, immune functioning, and brain functioning. Your microbiome can be harmed using antibiotics, illness, prolonged stress, aging, poor dietary habits, and unhealthy lifestyle choices. An imbalance of the microbial community in your gut can cause chronic diseases, obesity, and cancer. Research has also linked poor gut microbiome health to decreased energy, increased aggression, sleep challenges, communication challenges, and decreased social engagement in autistic individuals. Dietary components that support a healthy gut microbiome include probiotics, prebiotics, synbiotics, postbiotics, dairy products, spices (such as curcumin), and fruits and vegetables. The health of your gut microbiome is important and testable. Maybe testing your microbiome is your next action step?

Your poop tells you all about how your body feels about your food choices and how many nutrients you are absorbing from the food you are eating. Using the Bristol Stool Chart, you can determine if you need to eat foods that make your stool more stuck together or looser. Poop types three and four are good indicators that you are absorbing nutrients from your food. If your poop is hard and separate pellets, eating more mixed fruit and berries, live-culture yogurt, whole grains, seeds, beans, and legumes, along with drinking water or prune juice, will help balance your body. On the other hand, if your poop is closer to diarrhea, some bananas, apple sauce, dairy products, whole bread, pasta, rice, cooked carrots, and potatoes will support your digestion and overall health.

What does your poop tell you about what *your* body needs?

Nutrition Practice Reflections:

- What does your nutrition practice currently look like?
- What times of day do you typically eat?
- What feelings and sensations do you notice while eating?

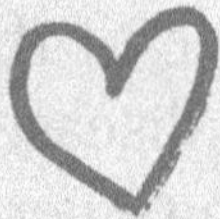

Nutrition Practice Reflections (continued):

- ✦ What feelings and sensations do you notice after eating?
- ✦ What shifts can you make to your sensory environment to support your nutrition practice?
- ✦ Does your nutrition practice recharge you enough?

Movement

"The key is figuring out which exercise you'll actually do. And I don't need scientific references for the notion that you are more likely to do a physical activity that you actually enjoy doing. It's a fundamental law of nature."

- Mark Sisson -

We are going to consider movement of two different types: daily movement within your routine and exercise as its own separate part of your schedule.

Movement throughout your day may be walking outside in the morning to check the mail, stretching while waiting at a red light, walking up and down the stairs, or standing up for computer breaks every so often. Simple tools can be game changers: setting alarms on your phone to remind you to get up, alternative seating options, a foam roller, or a stretch strap.

Exercise movement could be strength training or cardiovascular training or a combination. Physical challenges are a type of healthy stress, and every system in your body needs some stress in order to be its healthiest. Exercise movement can be a hard one for some people with a history of "should" and pressure from society to look a certain way, depending on your culture. The key is figuring out what kind of exercise you don't mind and maybe even enjoy.

When I started Polynesian dancing, my concept of exercise shifted. The combination of movement, music, and friendship made dance a type of exercise I look forward to! I had spent years trying to convince my body that I liked to run, and it turns out I just really don't. My parents are both amazing runners, and they love it: running makes them feel whole and regulated. I remember my mom talking about how she would pretend to be a deer and describe the lightness she felt training in college. Not me. But dancing or surfing? Yes please.

Your exercise movement preferences will depend on your sensory preferences. How does it feel to have sweat dripping down your skin? Does that sensation on a cardio machine at the gym under a fan match your preferences? How about squeezing into a wetsuit to swim in cold water or sliding on cowboy boots to country line dance? Your sensory preferences may not keep you from doing something, but they will likely influence your experience and how often you choose to do a certain type of exercise.

We all know exercise is good for you—no controversy there. But what does the research say about the impact of movement on your overall well-being? Exercise reduces the risk of some types of cancer, type-2 diabetes, and cardiovascular disease. The neuroscience of movement is compelling as well: decreasing depression symptoms; improving learning, executive functioning, and memory; and increasing neuroplasticity. Even the speed of areas in the brain communicating with each other increases with exercise! Exercise also shifts the way your brain processes dopamine, making it more available to support brain activity.

When considering exercise movement options, think about the people part: connection can be the key to helping you through the process of creating a habit. I mostly make it to the gym because one of my best friends is meeting me there. Bonus—two pillars of health in one!

Also consider your goals for your future. I want to be physically capable of scooping ice cream for my grandkids. What do you want your life to look like in five to ten years? Chances are some exercise will help you get there. So, let's do this!

With some extra motivation added in from the science, connection with others, and the encouragement of your future self, consider the time of day that fits your routine, roles, and energy level. Early morning? Mid-day? Evening? What can you build into your routine to help it happen? When I know my coffee is going to automatically brew at 5:00 AM, I get out of bed, and before I know it, I'm in my workout clothes and driving to the gym while sipping my coffee. Exercise movement is worth the effort, impacting heart health, breathing health, your immune system, endurance, strength, and mental health.

"At every level, from the microcellular to the psychological, exercise not only wards off the ill effects of chronic stress; it can also reverse them."

- John J. Ratey -

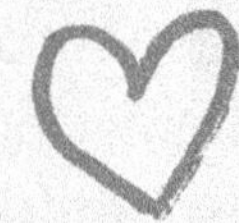

Movement Practice Reflections:

- What does your movement practice currently look like?
- Do you engage more often in exercise movement at a specific time of day or on certain days of the week?

Movement Practice Reflections: (continued):

- What feelings and sensations do you notice during your movement practice?
- What feelings and sensations do you notice after your movement practice?
- What shifts can you make to your sensory environment to support movement?
- Does your movement practice recharge you enough?

Connection

"I've learned that people will forget what you said, people will forget what you did, but people will never forget how you made them feel."

- Maya Angelou -

Whether you are an introvert or extrovert, you need some level and type of connection with others. We all need connection in our lives; it just might look different from one person to the next. Variables for connection time include how many people at one time, what activity, where, for how long, how often, and more. Think about how your sensory preferences impact your preferences for connection. Maybe you prefer a quieter space instead of a bustling coffee shop? Going for a walk instead of sitting?

The neuroscience research on connection is compelling! Social connection improves brain function, reducing the risk of cognitive decline and dementia and increasing resilience to the stress! The default mode network is activated and strengthened. We also see the release of the feel-good neurotransmitters, including oxytocin and dopamine, increasing well-being. Multiple studies show that being in a relationship, living with others, and weekly interactions with family and friends predict slower cognitive decline. Connection can protect against dementia and Alzheimer's. On the other hand, social pain, like being rejected, excluded, or betrayed, activates the same area of the brain (the anterior cingulate cortex) that is activated with physical pain. Research shows that social isolation is as much a risk factor for death as smoking and alcohol consumption. Connection is that important.

With a new understanding of your sensory preferences for connection but limited time, intentionally prioritize some time with people in your inner circle of friends and family. When you hang out with people you care about, turn off notifications that could alert your nervous system. Notice how you feel after spending time with each person you are close to. Tune into your body.

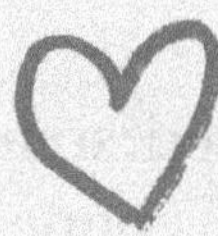

Connection Reflections:

- What does your connection time currently look like?
- Is there a time of day or are there certain days of the week when you more often connect with others?
- What feelings and sensations do you notice when you connect with others?
- What shifts can you make to your sensory environment to support connection?
- Does your connection time and intentional interactions with others recharge you enough?

Chapter 14

Contemplative Practices

"What we plant in the soil of contemplation, we shall reap in the harvest of action."

- Meister Eckhart -

Core to your sensory wellness pillars of health, *contemplative practices* encompass prayer, mindfulness, and meditation. All can help cultivate inner wisdom, decrease anxiety, improve focus and attention, increase feelings of gratitude, and reduce stress. Additionally, these contemplative practices may lower blood pressure, reduce the risk of heart disease, and improve immune function.

The impact on the brain really captivates and inspires me! Neuroscience research shows that during a time of being fully present, your brain becomes more ready to make new connections, increasing neuroplasticity. The time following mindfulness and prayer is a period of fluidity and openness to new pathways in the brain, and this amazing discovery has been confirmed by two kinds of neuroimaging: electroencephalogram (EEG) and magnetic resonance imaging (MRI)! Contemplative practices help us move toward the ebb and flow of healthy fluctuations in our autonomic nervous system's stress and calm responses and also shift neurochemistry to facilitate health and wellness. Research using MRI even confirms that when people recovering from addiction pray and then look at drinking-related images, they have reduced cravings and increased activation of the default mode network when compared to those who read a newspaper and then look at the same images. Another study showed that prayer reduces the intensity and unpleasantness of pain, showing reduced activity in the frontoparietal control network!

Choose the type of contemplative practice that fits you. Types of prayer include scripted prayers that you read and those that you create describing what you are thinking about or feeling. Prayers praise, ask, confess, seek forgiveness, and offer gratitude with words, sounds, or silence. Mindfulness is the practice of paying attention to the present moment without judgment. When practicing mindfulness, you calmly observe your thoughts and feelings, accept them with compassion, and choose curiosity about them without trying to change them. *Non-sleep deep rest* (NSDR), also referred to as Yoga Nidra, is another option. NSDR is a form of meditation that also has powerful effects on the nervous system, increasing dopamine and mental energy.

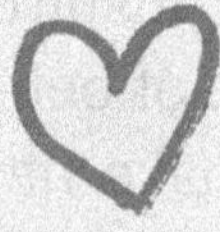

Contemplative Practice Reflections:

- ✦ What does your contemplative practice currently look like?
- ✦ Is there a time of day or are there certain days of the week when you more often engage in a contemplative practice?
- ✦ What feelings and sensations do you notice when you engage in a contemplative practice?
- ✦ What shifts can you make to your sensory environment to support a contemplative practice?
- ✦ Does your contemplative practice recharge you enough?

Chapter 14

Play & Leisure

"This is the real secret of life—to be completely engaged with what you are doing in the here and now. And instead of calling it work, realize it is play."

- Alan Watts -

What is your fun? In play, we allow ourselves to get lost in the present moment and enter into a flow of motivation, imagination, and full engagement. Our hearts feel more free, peaceful, content, joyful, and inspired. Play is powerful! Play builds resilience. Play supports connections in your brain and even the way your genes are expressed. Play increases curiosity. Play helps us navigate social connection. And play supports our physical health. These pillars of health are all connected!

What "counts" as play? Here are some of the elements that could be a part of your play:

- Play is intrinsically motivated: we don't play to get a reward; it is the reward and motivation in itself!
- Play is what you choose it to be and is not forced.
- Play is active, not happening to us or predetermined. There is no script.
- Play includes joyful discovery: a new game is created, adventures and treasures are found, and we learn new things!
- Play includes an element of imagination, allowing you to explore different worlds and possibilities.
- Play is joyful!

Does the concept of play still feel fuzzy? You are not alone. Many adults have a hard time coming up with leisure activities and then an even harder time prioritizing play. Here are some basic ideas to get your creative thoughts growing:

- Board games
- Team sports
- Painting
- Crafting
- Playing musical instruments
- Intimacy
- Dancing
- Hiking
- Storytelling
- Role-playing: acting classes or live action role-playing (LARPing)

There are so many options once you start brainstorming. When a client is feeling stuck in this area, I love talking through a leisure questionnaire or possible hobbies list and encouraging them to rate the hobbies based on how interested they are in trying each one (if they have never tried it) or doing it more (if they have done it and like it). For example: Sunrise photography! Have you ever tried it? If so, did you like it? If not, how interested are you in trying it? So many fun possibilities!

Vagus Nerve: The longest nerve in the body, connecting the brain to most of the major organs. The vagus nerve calms the body, helps with digestion, reduces inflammation, and manages other bodily functions.

In the midst of play, something very special happens in the nervous system. Through activation of the *ventral vagal complex*, a branch of the vagus nerve, the stress response and calm response happen at the same time. Remember the teeter totter from Chapter 1? It starts flying in the air instead of just moving up and down, one side and then the other! This unique activation of the autonomic nervous system, as described Dr. Stephen Porges in *The Pocket Guide to the Polyvagal Theory*, creates a safety zone where people can regulate their emotions and heal from trauma through play (2017). At the same time, your *default mode network*, *frontoparietal control network*, and *salience network* (a switch between the default mode network and the frontoparietal control network) are activated and enhanced (see more information about brain networks in the appendix). On the flip side, the lack of play can lead to depression and impede learning and social-emotional development.

"Through becoming familiar with play at the hands and hearts of thousands and thousands of children, I have learned that in any moment I have a choice—to fight, flee, or freeze, or to flow into connection. Such is the gift of play."

- Marc Otto -

Play is individual, personal, and most definitely multi-sensory. Play and leisure look different in every season of life, but in all seasons of life, play is not optional or frivolous. Play is key to sensory wellness.

"We don't stop playing because we grow old, we grow old because we stop playing."

- George Bernard Shaw -

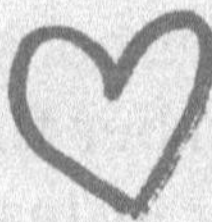

Play and Leisure Reflections:

- When do you remember last laughing?
- What is a fond memory of playing from your childhood?
- What does your play and leisure practice currently look like?
- Is there a time of day or certain days of the week when you play and participate in leisure activities more often?
- What feelings and sensations do you notice when you engage in play and leisure?
- What shifts can you make to your sensory environment to support play?
- Do your activities for fun and personal fulfillment recharge you enough?

How supportive is each pillar of health in helping you achieve your goals and meaningfully participate in what you want to prioritize? Where do you want to begin to grow more? Yes, all the multi-sensory pillars of health are important, vital to your well-being. But you can't change everything all at once. You can use the "Pillars of Health" resource in your *Sensory Wellness Reflection Journal* and on my website to help you decide what you want to change and in what order. Try focusing on one of the pillars of health and one concrete step forward in that area. Where do you want to start? Build momentum from there, adding in new shifts as you feel ready. Tell someone in your inner circle of connection about what you are working on and why. You got this!

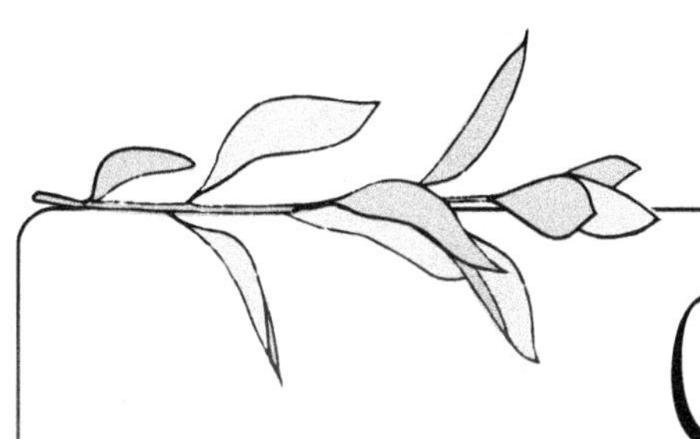

CHAPTER 15

Sensationally Me: Getting to Know More of Myself

"To know thyself is the beginning of wisdom."

~ Socrates ~

With the deeper understanding of your sensory preferences and a plan for your pillars of health, now is the time to renew the process of getting to know yourself in this season of life from a couple different angles. Use some of the tools and sensation shifts you discovered in the earlier chapters to bring alert and focused energy to the next concepts. Your senses will guide you as you lean into cultivating your core values, your roles, your decision process, and your response to stress.

Core Values

"Integrity is choosing courage over comfort; it's choosing what is right over what's fun, fast, or easy; and it's practicing your values, not just professing them."

~ Brené Brown ~

Grown into the fiber of your being are your values. Core values are the underlying principles you hold as most important. For some people, core values are conscious and intentional, rooted in your belief system, culture, role models, and/or the way you were raised. For others, your values are more informal and become clear through life events and how you give meaning to past experiences. Your values are part of your lens through which you sense everything happening around you. Inner peace and confidence grow out of getting more in touch with what matters most to you. More than this, research shows that awareness of core values and living in a way that aligns with them have amazing benefits:

- ✦ Enhanced authenticity
- ✦ Reduced stress and greater resilience
- ✦ Better decision-making and priority-setting
- ✦ Better attention to health
- ✦ Greater motivation, meaning, and goal fulfillment
- ✦ Improved relationship intimacy

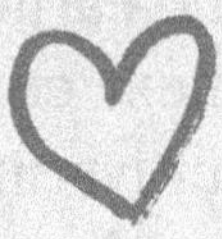

Living into your core values:

Do: Use the value cards in your *Sensory Wellness Reflection Journal* and on the website to sort the value cards into four piles: matters most, matters some, matters a little, does not matter to me. Tune into your internal senses as you consider each value. Then pare down the values that matter most to just three to five. These are your core values.

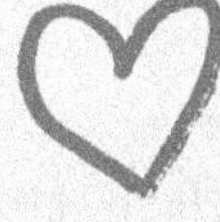

Living into your core values (continued):

Here are some questions to ask yourself to help:

- If I could only be _________ or _________, which would I choose?
- Consider the people you admire most. Are they more _________ or _________?
- Think back to the best and most painful moments you can remember. What do they show you about your core values?

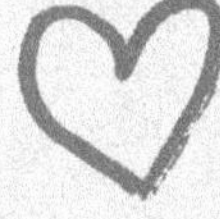

Reflect:

- What memory from your past aligns with your core values?
  - What did that memory look like?
  - Sound like?
  - Smell like?
  - Taste like?
  - Feel like?
  - How was your body positioned?
  - How were you moving?
  - What do you remember noticing in your body?
- Who knows your core values and encourages you to live into them?
- If no one does, who is a safe person you can share them with?

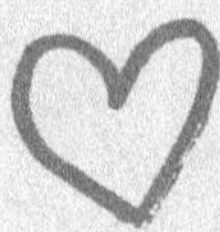

Reflect (continued):

- ✦ What are your early warning indicators your actions are not aligned with your values?
- ✦ What does it feel like when you are living aligned with your values?

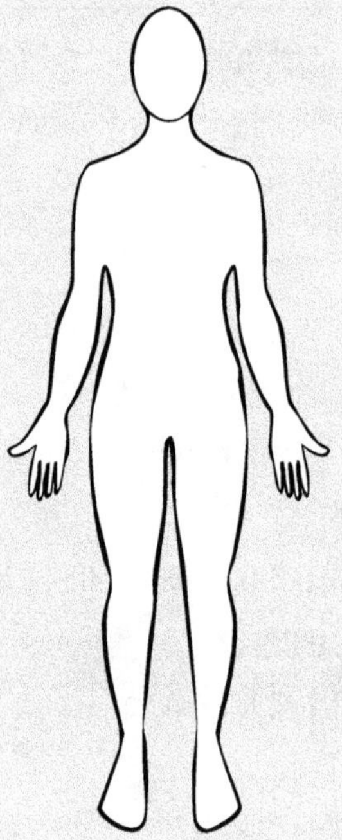

Your Roles

"The depth of your why determines the length of your what."

- Drew Sodestrom, Vintage Grace -

We are so much more than our routine activities and to-do lists. Much of the time, our roles in life give us purpose and meaning. We do not *find* meaning; we *make* meaning through all our multi-sensory life experiences. Meaning sustains us on the hard parts of our journeys, reassuring us we are a part of something much larger than ourselves.

While people have found meaning in many ways, three common sources of meaning are pursuing goals that leave an impact, a spiritual calling, and/or loving connections with others. Most of us will leave our greatest legacy through the people we interact with.

Prioritizing your roles:

Reflect:

- What are your roles in life in this season?
  Using the "My Roles" resource in the *Sensory Wellness Reflection Journal* and on the website, sort your current roles in life. Put the most important in the inner circle with your core values and work out from there, with the role that is least important to you on the outside ring.
- Look up your company's mission and vision statements. Do any words or concepts specifically capture your attention? How do the mission and vision statements overlap with and align with your core values?
- If you are a home and/or family operation manager, think about how your values impact your roles as a caregiver, partner, or volunteer.

Your Decision Process

"Between stimulus and response there is a space.
In that space is our power to choose our response.
In our response lies our growth and our freedom."

- Stephen Covey -

As you intentionally make decisions to prioritize the roles that matter most and your core values, you can shift out of reacting to life circumstances and move toward choosing to respond. The first step in this process is creating space between what happens and your actions.

For example, when I hear the sound of glass breaking and my children are nearby, my senses go into detective mode, gathering as much information as quickly as possible. My brain sorts through the emotions that flow through me as I run downstairs to investigate further.

It's like a *Choose Your Own Adventure* book, and I can choose how to handle the situation! I can either parent the broken glass situation in a reacting way, which may include dishing out consequences quickly and likely some yelling, or I can parent it in a responding way, which still means moving fast to make sure everyone is safe. However, responding instead of reacting includes a pause of however long it takes to consider how my core values impact my next move on the parenting front.

The first win and step of progress in your response in various situations is the pause: the opportunity to get to know yourself in a new or familiar situation. Bringing awareness to what you are sensing can help with the pause. If you create enough space between what happened and your response, you can flourish!

Reacting: Actions are automatic and often unconscious, triggered by past experiences, habits, or impulses.

Responding: Actions are thoughtful and intentional, allowing for conscious consideration and critical thinking.

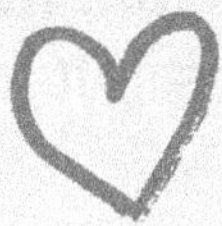

Refining your decision process:

Do: Once you practice pausing and responding instead of reacting, try an activity to help you make a decision and choose the best next step that is aligned with your most authentic self. The Decision Grid, Core Values Considerations, and/or Sense Experiment (in your *Sensory Wellness Reflection Journal*) can help you with intentional decision-making. You can use these tools for big decisions and small ones.

Reflect: Who has helped you be true to your core values in the way you respond, and as Mr. Rogers said, "helped you love the good that grows within you"? Send them a quick text and let them know, sharing gratitude for who they are in your life.

Your Response to Stress

Stressors can be a special gift in your garden of life. As the hard elements of life keep coming, we get the opportunity to check in on our why: our core values. We are invited to see how our values are influencing our daily lives and our responses to people in our lives. We don't become who we are meant to be without some challenges, and sometimes the hard can feel overwhelming. Stress deepens our why and grows our what.

Sitting in a meeting for one of my children's Individualized Education Program (IEP) meetings, I felt the importance of being deeply rooted in my why. Teachers, therapists, and administrators who cared deeply for my child reported to the group the areas where my child was doing well and the areas that still needed improvement. I could feel my body tensing up as the team discussed removing some of the therapy support to help improve my child's lisp. My heart reminded me: you have time to weigh out your options and decisions, but for now, just share your concerns and your why.

My concerns? Where to even begin? So complicated and yet so simple. I want my child to live and love fully, not hindered or impeded by a speech difference. That's why I'm here. How do you write that into an IEP? As my regulation arousal level increased, I took a slow, deep breath and shared my thoughts with the team. I was assertive, kind, and intentional. As I opened up, the IEP team members emotionally and physically leaned in. We were working together, in sync.

Moving Through the Stress Cycle

In Emily and Amelia Nagoski's book, *Burnout*, they point out, "Just because you've dealt with the stressor doesn't mean you've dealt with the stress itself" (2020). When sensation comes in strong and overwhelming, the sensation can be a stressor all by itself, separate from what is happening: the intense sound waves in addition to the person yelling. This creates even more urgency in processing through your lid flipping and moving that influx of stress through your body and out. You are not only working through the situational stressor, but also the sensory and physiological stress at the same time.

Dealing with the situational stressor (the storm of deciding what school will be best for your child or how to pay for the therapy your child very much needs) is a separate process from working through and completing what the Nagoskis call "the stress cycle" in your body.

Remember the section on the fight, flight, freeze, or flock responses when your sympathetic nervous system activation skyrockets (see page 3)? Completing the stress cycle is a crucial component of cleaning up after the storm physiologically and decreasing the cortisol levels in your body so you can be ready for what life brings next.

Stress is not bad; it is just supposed to not be around all the time, every day, day in and day out. Stressors can help us choose the right path, have energy to do hard things, and clarify our values and purpose. We work with stress to these ends by opening up to and being aware of the sensation that comes with the stressor. When we block or numb the sensations and emotions, we fight against the stress and suffer the adverse effects on our bodies and our minds.

That stressful afternoon, I finished the IEP meeting and went home. Time for more coffee, just decaf this time. As I brewed the coffee, I could feel the tension in my neck and upper back. My breath was shallow, and my heartbeat was on the quicker side. The cars driving by sounded louder than I remembered, and my dog's barking was grating on my nerves more than normal. I lay down on the floor, slowly contracting muscle groups and relaxing them. I moved into yoga's child pose and then downward dog, alternating pushing each heel into the ground. Twenty minutes later, as I slowly sipped my dark roast coffee, swirled with milk, I felt more ready to move on to the next part of my day: work meetings.

"Over the years you realize one of the best things you can do is become a safe place for yourself."

- Stacie Martin -

You cannot positive-self-talk yourself out of the stress response. You move through it, literally, with muscle contractions and movement. Keys to moving on and completing the stress cycle? Proprioceptive (*muscles and joints*) and vestibular (*movement*) sensations. The internal senses help you navigate life's storms, and you don't have to go to the gym and do official "exercise."

Laughter works, as you contract many muscles by laughing. I used to get home from a stress-filled day and turn on an old episode of *Candid Camera* to complete the stress cycle, but I didn't know that was what I was doing. For whatever reason, that show just cracks me up and helps my body to process both the stressors of the day and the stress within my body. Do you have a favorite comedian? *Saturday Night Live* skit? Dad joke?

Crying works too! While not as fun as laughing so hard you get a side ache, crying releases the cortisol and completes the stress cycle as well. Have you ever felt better after a good cry?

Here are some ways to move the stress through your body:

- Twenty-plus minutes of physical activity
- Progressive muscle contraction and relaxation
- Breathing techniques
- Positive social interaction
- Laughter
- Affection
- A big cry
- Creative expression

Your Response to Stress:

Do: Which one of the stress movers will you try today?

Reflect: Think of a time when you felt stressed. Once the stressor was gone, what did you feel in your body?

- ✦ What did that memory look like?
- ✦ Sound like?
- ✦ Smell like?
- ✦ Taste like?
- ✦ Feel like?
- ✦ How was your body positioned?
- ✦ How were you moving?
- ✦ What do you remember noticing in your body?

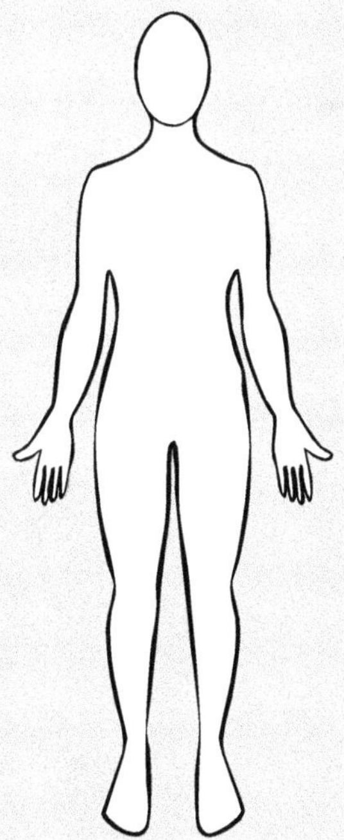

Prevent stress from being a barrier to leaning into who you truly are and helping you get to know yourself more. You are not your stress, and yet, often, people see how you respond to stress and assume who you must be. So, for yourself and for others, move through stress and navigate the stressors in ways that intentionally align with your core values.

Getting to know yourself continues unfolding throughout your seasons of life. You are sensationally unique with every fiber of your being, every sensory receptor. You are on purpose and for a purpose. The world is a better place every day you show up, fully and sensationally you!

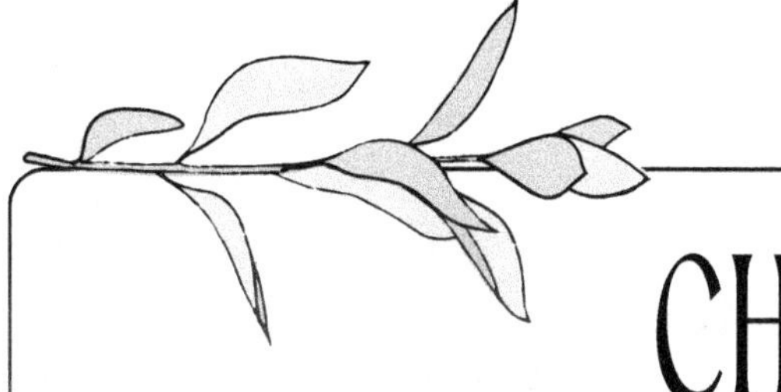

CHAPTER 16

Sensory Wellness in Relationships: At Home and at Work

"When someone truly can be trusted to see who you are and want what's best for you, no matter your official relationship, they are family."

- Oprah Winfrey -

Whether we are at work or at home, healthy relationships are key to our overall sensory wellness. We were made to live in community. People can help us thrive and feel like sunshine on a spring day. Or our relationships with others can tear us down and life can start to feel too hard. How do we bring our best selves into interactions, staying true to our values and honoring our own journeys? Relationship is back and forth communication at its core: full-body, multi-sensory communication. How can we communicate well in order to build respectful and trusting relationships?

Internal Sense Communication: Tuning into Your Interoceptive Sensations to Communicate

The foundation of relationships, both at work and at home, is our communication with ourselves. Think of all the expressions about our body communicating with us!

"I had a gut feeling."
"My heart sank."
"A knot in my stomach."
"Butterflies in my stomach."
"A prickly sensation."
"My skin crawled."
"A sinking feeling in my body."
"A chill down my spine."
"My intuition was telling me."
"My body was sending me signals."

These expressions, while not necessarily literal, focus on body sensations, a physical feeling that is often associated with an unexplainable inner knowing or intuition. I call this *internal sense communication*. Your communication with your own body can tell you both positive and negative things. Depending on the situation, these body messages can indicate like, dislike, and an array of emotions. The inner senses will guide you in relationships.

"Your body is a messenger
A web of connection
A key to resistance
A well of resources
A soft place to land
An invitation to be here now"

- Hillary McBride -

I recently had a huge full-body reaction where it felt like my body was yelling at me. An older teen I mentor wanted to talk with me about something they were struggling with: the realization of a codependent relationship. As they described the situation, I could feel my legs start to shake, not noticeably to anyone else, just little micromovements back and forth. My palms were sweaty, and my heart rate kicked up more than a couple of notches. The teen shared, and I showed up for them: holding the space, reflecting and validating, being with them. When the conversation ended and they went home, I sat bewildered. What was my body telling me? I spent time journaling and exploring what I felt, being there with—and for—myself. Through this tuning into my inner senses, I realized some thoughts I wanted to share with this teen, and our relationship deepened because of these insights. When journaling and tuning into my body, I also connected the dots of how their situation brought me back to a situation from my past. I could empathize deeply because of my own struggle with codependency.

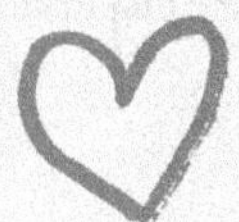

Reflect: When did your internal senses guide you in an interaction recently? What did you notice in your body?

External Sense Communication: Tuning into Your Exteroceptive Sensations to Communicate

Communication is most effective when we use all our senses, including our exteroceptive input, to understand. You may notice the way the corners of a person's lips are turning upward and infer they are smiling. You may hear a lowered tone in a person's voice. You may feel their gentle touch and hear their words with a more nurturing and loving tone.

A person's posture tells you a lot about the meaning behind their words. A research study showed that people do a better job of guessing the emotion a person is experiencing if they get to observe the person's body cues than if they just get to see the person's facial expression. External sense communication also gathers information from the environment. Is it raining? Scorching hot? Are thunder clouds rolling in? These clues give context to the information so that the brain can do its best job of making sense of the interaction, predicting what might happen next, and deciding what to do or say next. We need all the external sense information to communicate clearly and kindly.

Reflect: When did your external senses guide you in an interaction recently? What did you notice around you?

Emotions

"I remember the first time I understood as an adult that my body was saying something worth listening to, something that deserved to be heard."

- Hillary L. McBride -

As we move from communication toward relationships, let's take some time to think about emotions. Emotions have the power to connect us for a lifetime or put a wall between people that can divide families for generations and hurt many people along the way. Emotions are powerful, but they don't need to have power over us. I like thinking of emotions as consultants, almost like how my dad used to call me his copilot when we drove somewhere. I was in charge of giving suggestions about routes, changing the music, opening food containers for him, and sometimes making sure he was paying attention to the road construction ahead as he sang songs from the Temptations with all the passion of a true performer. I wasn't the one driving. What emotions tell us is relevant and helpful, but they don't get to drive, and they also do not just disappear or go away if we ignore them. We get to learn to be with them, determine how they were constructed, and not kick them out of the car.

Emotions are not a set group of feelings we are born with, nor are they even the same from one person to the next. New neuroscience research on emotions by Lisa Feldman Barrett and her team, amongst other scientists, shows that emotions are not just passively reacted to, they are actively constructed (2017). Constructed from a combination of past experiences, concepts, and sensation, emotions predict and categorize sensory information every moment through an active process you can change.

"Emotions that seem to happen to you are made by you."

- Lisa Feldman Barrett -

What role do past experiences have in constructing emotions? Past experiences can be split into implicit memories and explicit memories. Both impact the process of making emotions. Both implicit and explicit memories are encoded or filed away in your brain in similar regions, with each person's brain's memory process varying slightly. However, the retrieval of these memories happens in different areas of the brain.

Implicit memories start to form before you are born as you attune to your biological mother's heartbeat when you perceive different sensations. These memories are created unconsciously based on what is happening around you and what you are experiencing. For instance, if, as you were growing up, your family had people over for dinner all the time and you watched your parents laughing and having fun connecting with new and old friends, you likely have implicit memories that help your brain unconsciously predict that if people are coming over, it will bring joy and excitement. Implicit memories also help you unconsciously decide what is familiar and therefore deeply coded as probably safe. If you and your family interacted with lots of people of different ethnicities and socioeconomic backgrounds while you were growing up, you will likely have a lower physiologic arousal level if a person who has a different skin tone or cultural background starts talking to you at the park. This is not a conscious decision or how your body has to stay during the interaction, but it is your body's knee-jerk response based on implicit memories. Implicit memories also help you develop skills like riding a bike or folding clothes. Interestingly, trauma experiences can be encoded and stored in the brain as implicit memories, determining your physical and emotional response to sensation before you have a conscious thought about the loud sound you just heard or the taste of the food during a meal. Implicit memories are encoded or filed in many brain systems, including the same one that is known for motor coordination, thinking, and emotional processing!

Explicit memories are details of facts and events, including personal experiences and general knowledge that is not autobiographical that you recall consciously. You search your mind for a memory from your childhood, recalling a specific date or conversation. Or you memorize math facts and then quickly add numbers together at the grocery store using those math facts. Explicit memories can fade over time or stay vivid in your mind. Explicit memories are stored throughout your brain and begin their journey of being filed in the medial temporal lobe. When personal experience memories are recalled, you are using the *frontoparietal control network*, known for goal-directed control processes, and the *default mode network*, known as the key network in self-reflection.

"Emotions are not reactions to the world. You are not a passive receiver of sensory input but an active constructor of your emotions. From sensory input and past experience, your brain constructs meaning and prescribes action."

- Lisa Feldman Barrett -

As Feldman Barrett points out, simple feelings are different from constructed emotions and are hard-wired when you are born. They are a summary of what is going on inside you physiologically: calmness, agitation, excitement, comfort, and discomfort. These feelings lack detail and need meaning, past experiences, and context to be added.

In the book *Practices for Embodied Living*, Hillary McBride details how emotions can help us by predicting meaning and inspiring us to action (2024). In the last decade, I learned that emotions are neither good nor bad. We may enjoy some of them more than others, and they are all helpful. Now I am grateful for each of them, most of the time.

"FEAR makes us alert, detects threat, and helps us get away from danger
SADNESS helps us encounter what is meaningful, signals that we need care or rest, and helps us grieve
JOY helps us expand, heal, celebrate, connect, and share
DISGUST protects us from what is toxic to our bodily or social systems
EXCITEMENT gives us motivation, creates energy, and helps us explore and investigate
ANGER asserts, protects, defends, or helps us make change
DESIRE helps us get pleasure, identify wants, meet needs, and create"

- Hillary McBride -

In my 30's, I decided to not be afraid of emotions or surfing in the same season of life. I don't know why I was afraid of emotions. I had loving parents who encouraged me to use "I feel" statements before that was even a thing. Nothing majorly traumatizing happened to me, but I did put a lot of pressure on myself to succeed. I'm still a recovering perfectionist. But somewhere along the way, I decided I didn't like emotions, and because I felt out of control, I stuffed emotions down instead of letting them copilot.

So there I was, going through one of the hardest seasons of my life up to that point. At home, interactions with my husband were rough. Then at work, a therapist would quit, be hit by a client, or feel down about life. A family would be going through the depths of trying to understand who they had imagined their child would be and grappling with who their child really is. Best case, acceptance. Hardest to watch: a parent trying to change their child more than help them. The child left way, way over-scheduled, miserable, and feeling like they were broken, invisible, or, worse, bad. I used to picture myself symbolically standing on the shore of life with my surfboard under my arm, getting knocked down by the waves. I couldn't even get my feet underneath me before the next wave would hit.

But then, I did my own therapy with a wonderful counselor, processing my past, accepting my present, and not getting myself all riled up about the future. I realized that I could not and did not want to control all aspects of my life. As I settled into the process, I found that I could stand in the waves.

I could sit with people in their hard season of life without feeling knocked over by their wave. I could empathize, "You have had a bad day? I am here for you, to sit with you in the dark. That must be terrible. Sounds like you are feeling so hurt, devastated."

The waves still crashed, but my footing got stronger. And then I felt a stirring: surfing. It was calling to me. I would think about it randomly. I had taken a couple of lessons almost twenty years before. Three kids and a lot less abdominal strength later, surfing? And yet the stirring continued, would come up at odd times, and didn't go away. And then some friends heard about all the hard things I was going through and invited me away for a girls' weekend: *surfing!* I said yes and felt like God was listening, answering my deepest heart stirrings when I hadn't even given them words.

My excitement grew and grew. The night before I was going to take a surf lesson, I was so nervous. I asked for a pep talk. Tell me the language, the culture, the rules. What do I do? Wear? How do I move? My friends talked me through it, complete with what to do in case of a shark attack.

That morning, I started to realize what was happening. I cried. I was moving from standing in the waves of life to riding them (or trying to). There were still waves. But I was going to dance with them, paint lines in the water with the movement of my surfboard as the waves moved me. I was actively getting into position to catch them. I was paddling hard. I was popping up and balancing (sometimes). I was riding the waves! My surf coach told me there is nothing like feeling the power of the wave moving you as you dance with it. Yes! An active process, not just happening to me. No more waves crashing on me as I just stand on the shore. I am in the ocean now, actively lining up for the wave and going for it!

That first day had a lot of falling into the waves and being tossed around. I kept paddling until I was mentally and physically exhausted. The adrenaline had worn off, and my body felt limp. I stayed out in the waves and felt them swell under me. I watched the horizon and saw the vastness of God's love. I smiled so big as I watched my friends and coach catch waves. There are waves for everyone. I caught a couple more and felt a new sense of calm. It has taken time to learn to ride the waves, but the point of that first day was to move off the symbolic shore of my life and out of the shore break, where waves repeatedly crash. To have the courage to ride the waves of emotions.

The wave of emotion is powerful! At first, sensation arises, like a hill of water on the horizon. Sensation builds as the water rises, and there is a peak of sensational intensity. The water starts to crash, and sometimes we feel a second reaction of defense or insight about what to do next. After we ride the wave of emotion, we may feel satisfaction, relief, and awe. We store the memory away to help us give meaning to future situations and feelings, communicating and connecting with ourselves and sometimes others. Now we know that we don't just get to choose which wave of emotion we want to surf, we get to make our own waves.

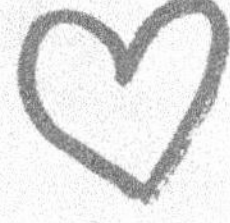

Tuning into Emotions:

Reflect:

- What emotions have been helpful copilots recently?
- When did you let emotions "drive" recently?

Do: Connect with a trustworthy friend or partner. Use the Experiences and Emotions wheel in your *Sensory Wellness Reflection Journal.* Take turns being the sharing person and the listener. The person sharing says, "I felt _____ (describe the sensation and choose an emotion from the feelings wheel), when _________ (describe a situation briefly)," for a couple of emotions. The listener's job is to acknowledge, not fix or offer advice, with sounds like "mmm" or "ohhh" or nodding their head, and then at the end say, "Thank you for sharing all that." Then switch. How did it feel to share? How did it feel to listen?

Building Relationships Rooted in Sensory Wellness

Relationships, at home and at work, are strengthened by repeated interactions that show a person to be trustworthy. We are trustworthy when we are aware of our sensory and emotional regulation and their potential impact on the interaction. Once you are aware of what is happening with your own processing of sensory information and your emotions, how can you interact with someone you care about in a trustworthy, present way? Empathy.

Empathy is a trustworthiness booster and is very different from sympathy. Empathy fuels connection, while sympathy drives disconnection. Theresa Wiseman, a nursing scholar, determined empathy has four qualities:

- ✦ Perspective taking
- ✦ Staying out of judgment
- ✦ Recognizing emotion in others
- ✦ Communicating back the emotion you see

Empathy sounds like:

- ✦ "What I hear you saying is ________."
- ✦ "Sounds like ________."
- ✦ So ________ (repeat what you heard). What did I miss?"

In the book, *Daring Greatly*, Brené Brown describes empathy as showing someone they are not alone, which can be hard because it forces us to connect with the parts of ourselves that know that feeling, the multi-sensory memories that encompass similar emotions (2015). It is not saying things like the following:

- ✦ "Must be hard to be you."
- ✦ "Well at least ________."
- ✦ "Here's some advice."

Empathy is being with the person who is in the hard situation. Being with, not doing something for. It's holding up a mirror and showing them: I see you and I hear you.

One year, our clinical team focused on empathy as the theme for the year, and we talked about reflecting back emotions. We found an organization that helps women escape sex trafficking and choose a career that allows them to do something different. These women were making beautiful necklaces from recycled metal mirrors they'd cut into circles. Then they took recycled metal and folded it around the mirror and then made beads with recycled paper. I bought them for our whole team and told the therapists, "This mirror is your best friend. It reminds you that you don't have to fix it or change the reflection in the mirror when you empathize. You also don't have to let someone else's struggle soak into you and become yours to carry. You can say what Brené Brown taught me, "I don't even know what to say, but I'm so glad that you told me. It sounds like you just went through something really hard." I like to call that necklace my "empathy shield," and I still wear it because, as a mom and a helping professional, I see and hear about a lot of hard situations and experiences that I want to bring empathy to, but I don't want to get burnt out because I am carrying everyone's challenges.

Reflect: When have you felt your body resisting or pulling away from an empathy moment? Why do you think that particular situation was hard? That empathy opportunity may have given you the gift of showing you a place where you have a wound or hurt from the past that you are now ready to heal.

Empathy can be hard enough when you are listening to someone you care about go through something rough. But what about when someone you care about has been hurt *by you*, and they are bringing it *to you* to tell you about how they were hurt so you can work together to repair the relationship? This can be an even harder level of empathy.

Our goal in a situation where someone's "hard" has to do with you is to be present. Staying within a connected, respectful zone while you are communicating with the person can be difficult. It can feel tempting to withdraw or communicate passively, aggressively, or passive-aggressively. Choosing to listen, reflect, and validate grows the relationship and builds trust.

"Don't shrink. Don't puff up. Stand your sacred ground."

- Brené Brown -

Have you ever noticed yourself reacting by getting smaller: underestimating something exciting, talking quieter or less, or even rounding your shoulders and standing shorter? Or puffing up: overexaggerating something so you look more amazing or braver, talking louder and more, or pushing out your chest like a peacock displaying its brilliant feathers? When I heard Brené Brown describe these types of interactions, my eyes were opened to another component of self-awareness in interactions. Am I making myself sound more or less smart, more or less busy, different from the real me? If so, why? Is something happening sensory-wise in me or around me that is shifting me from being my true self? Is there an emotion forming, rooted in something that happened to me or around me, that is influencing how I am showing up? My sensational body is trying to have a conversation with me. What is it saying?

Reflect: When have you puffed up or gotten smaller in a situation? What do you think was happening inside and around you that shifted you away from your sacred ground and true self?

When a person reaches out to let you know that they felt hurt by something you did or said, you can start by reflecting back what you heard. You can also say, "Help me understand this better." If you are unsure if you are ready to be present in this feedback type of situation, check in with your senses. You can tell the person you need a little time before connecting about what hurt them because you want to listen well and understand. Let them know you will reach out to tell them as soon as you are ready. It is more than okay to pause a conversation; that pause is respectful and kind. Just make sure you do circle back.

Here are sensory reflection questions to see if you are ready:

- **Ears:** Am I ready to listen and not interrupt?
- **Mouth:** Am I ready to ask curious questions and recognize the person's strengths?
- **Eyes:** Am I ready to see the person and not avoid looking in their direction? Am I ready to see the problem as separate from the person?
- **Skin:** Do I feel flushed? Are my palms sweaty?
- **Body position:** Do I feel ready to sit next to the person? Are any of my muscles clenched?
- **Interoceptive:** What is my breathing like? How fast is my heart beating?

Sensory wellness in relationships looks like self-awareness that leads to emotional fluidity and agency. Emotional fluidity and agency give birth to empathy that supports you staying true to yourself while connecting with others in thriving relationships.

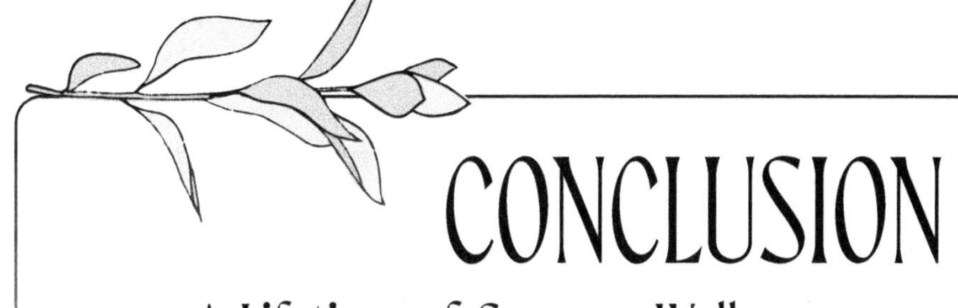

CONCLUSION

A Lifetime of Sensory Wellness

"Forever is composed of nows."

- Emily Dickinson -

Sensory wellness is the ebb and flow throughout each day and season of life. Health is movement in all aspects of our being.

Breathe in, breathe out.
Increase heart rate, decrease heart rate.
Influence internal and external sensation, determine meaning.
Activate stress response, activate calm response.
Increase energy level, decrease energy level.
Ride waves of emotion, float on calm waters of pause.
Respond, adjust.
Change, accept.
Connect with others, connect with myself.
As we go...as we are...this is sensory wellness.

You soak in the rays of sunshine. You extend roots of strength. You sway in the breeze. You drink in the sweet rain of spring. This is you growing strong, flourishing. Being open to changes over time, you welcome the evolution of your senses throughout your lifetime, thriving in all seasons of life.

It is an honor to travel together on this journey. While not often a straight path, the journey of loving well is worth it. You are worth it. Remember to be patient with yourself. Adjustments take time, new routines and habits require intentionality and energy to grow. When life doesn't go as you were hoping, be generous with forgiveness and search for the door of a new opportunity opening. As you continue to learn, explore, and cultivate different areas of your life, I hope you and your loved ones come back to the reflection questions in this book to illuminate your path as guides for thriving. Let's all continue writing our stories of working through challenges and thriving. I hope *Sensory Wellness* is just a new beginning for you.

Until we meet again,
I hope you savor the joy of your sensational life.

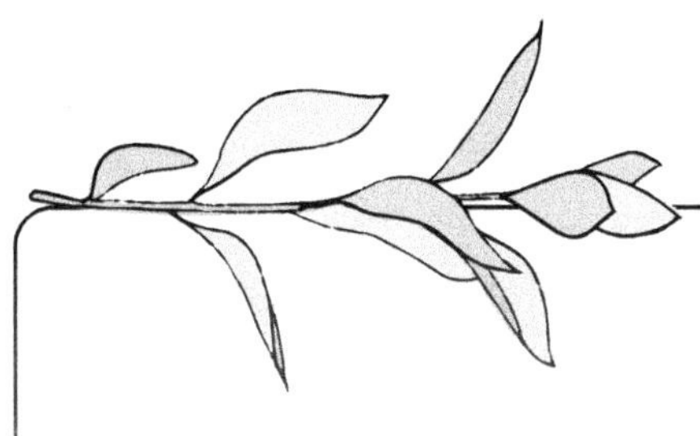

APPENDIX

Understanding The Neuroscience Research: The Yeo Seven Network Brain Model

The Yeo Seven Network Model is a widely used grouping of coordinated networks in the brain that shows how brain regions work together. Neuroscience research reveals insights about brain connection patterns and helps us learn more about sensory integration and processing, the pillars of health, and how to thrive. Here is a list of the brain networks, the areas of the brain each network connects, the function of each network, and examples of that network in action in daily life.

1. **Visual Network (VN)**
   - **Location:** Primarily in the occipital lobe (back of the brain).
   - **Function:** Processes visual information—shapes, colors, motion, spatial layout.
   - **Example:** Reading text, recognizing faces, navigating a room.

2. **Somatomotor Network (SMN)**
   - **Location:** Precentral gyrus (primary motor cortex), postcentral gyrus (primary somatosensory cortex), supplementary motor areas.
   - **Function:** Movement control and body sensation.

- **Example:** Moving your hand, feeling temperature, coordinating speech muscles.

3. **Dorsal Attention Network (DAN)**
   - **Location:** Includes frontal eye fields, intraparietal sulcus, superior parietal lobule.
   - **Function:** Top-down, goal-directed attention—selecting stimuli relevant to a task.
   - **Example:** Searching for a friend in a crowd, following a moving object.

4. **Ventral Attention Network (VAN)**
   - **Location:** Temporoparietal junction, ventral frontal cortex.
   - **Function:** Bottom-up attention—detecting unexpected or salient events.
   - **Example:** Suddenly noticing a flashing light or someone calling your name.

5. **Limbic Network**
   - **Location:** Orbitofrontal cortex, temporal pole, parts of medial temporal lobe.
   - **Function:** Emotion, memory, and motivation; strong connections with the hippocampus and amygdala.
   - **Example:** Feeling nostalgia when hearing an old song.

6. **Frontoparietal Control Network (FPN)**
   - **Location:** Lateral prefrontal cortex, inferior parietal lobule.
   - **Function:** Flexible cognitive control—integrating information from other networks to guide decisions.
   - **Example:** Planning your day, solving a new problem, switching between tasks.

7. **Default Mode Network (DMN)**
   - **Location:** Medial prefrontal cortex, posterior cingulate cortex/precuneus, angular gyrus.
   - **Function:** Self-referential thought, mind-wandering, autobiographical memory, theory of mind.
   - **Example:** Daydreaming, thinking about the future, remembering the past.

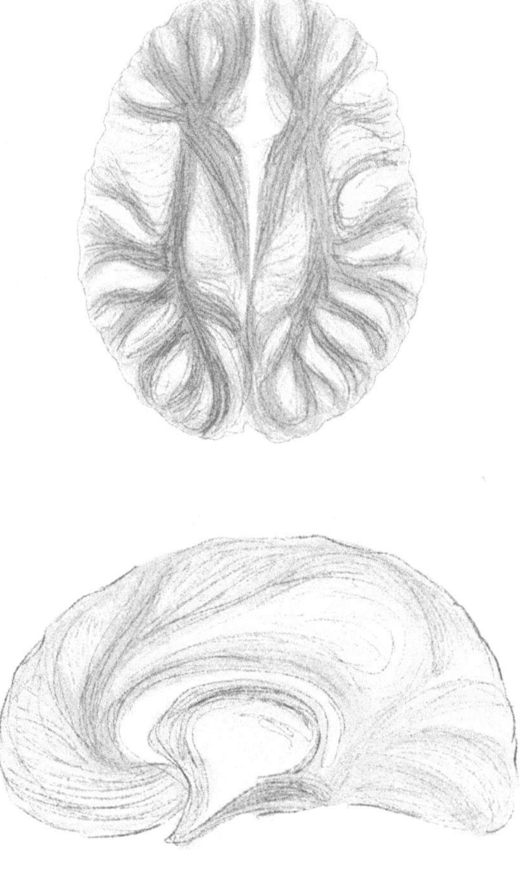

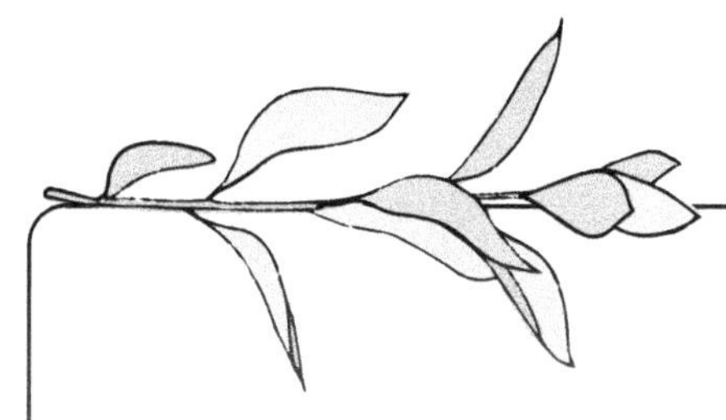

REFERENCES

Introduction Reference

Rabin, Karden. 2022. "Defining Embodiment." *Trauma Research Foundation*, September 27, 2022. https://traumaresearchfoundation.org/defining-embodiment/.

Chapter 1 References

Balint, Elisabeth Maria, Viktorija Daniele, Dominik Langgartner, Stefan O. Reber, Eva Rothermund, Harald Gündel, Jörn von Wietersheim, Thomas Buckley, and Marc N. Jarczok. 2023. "Heart Rate Variability Predicts Outcome of Short-Term Psychotherapy at the Workplace." *Psychophysiology* 60 (1): e14150. https://doi.org/10.1111/psyp.14150.

Benarroch, E. E. 2014. "Sympathetic System: Overview." In Encyclopedia of the Neurological Sciences, edited by Michael J. Aminoff and Robert B. Daroff, 2nd ed. Amsterdam: Elsevier. https://doi.org/10.1016/B978-0-12-385157-4.00514-5.

Benarroch, E. E. 2014. "Sympathetic System: Overview." In *Encyclopedia of the Neurological Sciences*, edited by Michael J. Aminoff and Robert B. Daroff, 2nd ed. Amsterdam: Elsevier. https://doi.org/10.1016/B978-0-12-385157-4.00514-5.

Dunne, Julie, Michael Flores, Richa Gawande, and Zev Schuman-Olivier. 2021. "Losing Trust in Body Sensations: Interoceptive Awareness and Depression Symptom Severity among Primary Care Patients." *Journal of Affective Disorders* 282 (March): 1–7. https://doi.org/10.1016/j.jad.2020.12.092.

Duquette, Patrice. 2017. "Increasing Our Insular World View: Interoception and Psychopathology for Psychotherapists." *Frontiers in Neuroscience* 11 (March): 135. https://doi.org/10.3389/fnins.2017.00135.

Fink, George, ed. 2010. *Encyclopedia of Stress*. 2nd ed. Amsterdam: Academic Press. https://doi.org/10.5860/choice.45-4131.

Geisler, Fay C. M., Nadja Vennewald, Thomas Kubiak, and Hannelore Weber. 2010. "The Impact of Heart Rate Variability on Subjective Well-Being Is Mediated by Emotion Regulation." *Personality and Individual Differences* 49 (7): 723–28. https://doi.org/10.1016/j.paid.2010.06.015.

Khalsa, Sahib S., Ralph Adolphs, Oliver G. Cameron, Hugo D. Critchley, Paul W. Davenport, Justin S. Feinstein, Jamie D. Feusner, et al. 2018. "Interoception and Mental Health: A Roadmap." *Biological Psychiatry: Cognitive Neuroscience and Neuroimaging* 3 (6, June): 501–13. https://doi.org/10.1016/j.bpsc.2017.12.004.

Kuniishi, Hiroshi, Yuko Nakatake, Masayuki Sekiguchi, and Mitsuhiko Yamada. 2022. "Adolescent Social Isolation Induces Distinct Changes in the Medial and Lateral OFC-BLA Synapse and Social and Emotional Alterations in Adult Mice." *Neuropsychopharmacology* 47 (9): 1641–52. https://doi.org/10.1038/s41386-022-01358-6.

Lalanza, Jaume F., Sonia Lorente, Raimon Bullich, Carlos García, Josep Maria Losilla, and Lluis Capdevila. 2023. "Methods for Heart Rate Variability Biofeedback (HRVB): A Systematic Review and Guidelines." *Applied Psychophysiology and Biofeedback* 48 (4): 365–83. https://doi.org/10.1007/s10484-023-09582-6.

Makovac, Elena, Sarah N. Garfinkel, Andrea Bassi, Barbara Basile, Emiliano Macaluso, Mara Cercignani, Giovanni Calcagnini, et al. 2015. "Effect of Parasympathetic Stimulation on Brain Activity during Appraisal of Fearful Expressions." *Neuropsychopharmacology* 40 (7): 1649–58. https://doi.org/10.1038/npp.2015.10.

Murphy, Jennifer, Rebecca Brewer, Caroline Catmur, and Geoffrey Bird. 2017. "Interoception and Psychopathology: A Developmental Neuroscience Perspective." *Developmental Cognitive Neuroscience* 24 (April): 45–54. https://doi.org/10.1016/j.dcn.2016.12.006.

Purves, D., G. J. Augustine, and D. Fitzpatrick. 2001. "Autonomic Regulation of Sexual Function." In *Neuroscience*, 2nd ed. Sunderland, MA: Sinauer Associates.

Schmitt, Carolyn M., and Sarah A. Schoen. 2022. "Interoception: A Multi-Sensory Foundation of Participation in Daily Life." *Frontiers in Neuroscience* 16 (April): 875200. https://doi.org/10.3389/fnins.2022.875200.

Shaffer, Fred, and J. P. Ginsberg. 2017. "An Overview of Heart Rate Variability Metrics and Norms." *Frontiers in Public Health* 5: 258. https://doi.org/10.3389/fpubh.2017.00258.

Siegel, Daniel J., and Tina Payne Bryson. 2011. *The Whole-Brain Child: 12 Revolutionary Strategies to Nurture Your Child's Developing Mind.* New York: Delacorte Press.

Winfrey, Oprah, and Bruce D. Perry. 2021. *What Happened to You: Conversations on Trauma, Resilience, and Healing.* New York: Flatiron Books.

Chapter 2 References

Chen, Wen G., Dana Schloesser, Angela M. Arensdorf, Janine M. Simmons, Changhai Cui, Rita Valentino, James W. Gnadt, et al. 2021. "The Emerging Science of

Interoception: Sensing, Integrating, Interpreting, and Regulating Signals within the Self." *Trends in Neurosciences* 44 (1, January): 3–16. https://doi.org/10.1016/j.tins.2020.10.007.

Couto, Blas, Federico Adolfi, Lucas Sedeño, Alejo Salles, Andrés Canales-Johnson, Pablo Alvarez-Abut, Indira Garcia-Cordero, et al. 2015. "Disentangling Interoception: Insights from Focal Strokes Affecting the Perception of External and Internal Milieus." *Frontiers in Psychology* 6 (May): 503. https://doi.org/10.3389/fpsyg.2015.00503.

Crucianelli, Laura, Adam Enmalm, and H. Henrik Ehrsson. 2022. "Interoception as Independent Cardiac, Thermosensory, Nociceptive, and Affective Touch Perceptual Submodalities." *Biological Psychology* 172: 108355. https://doi.org/10.1016/j.biopsycho.2022.108355.

Skrzypulec, Błażej. 2021. "Blur and Interoceptive Vision." *Philosophical Studies* 178 (10): 3331–47. https://doi.org/10.1007/s11098-021-01601-8.

Chapter 3 References

Kawamura, Satoru, and Shuji Tachibanaki. 2012. "Explaining the Functional Differences of Rods versus Cones." *Wiley Interdisciplinary Reviews: Membrane Transport and Signaling* 1 (5): 675–83. https://doi.org/10.1002/wmts.8

Siu, Caitlin R., and Kathryn M. Murphy. 2018. "The Development of Human Visual Cortex and Clinical Implications." *Eye and Brain* 10: 25–36. https://doi.org/10.2147/EB.S130893.

References

Chapter 4 References

Ekdale, Eric G. 2016. "Form and Function of the Mammalian Inner Ear." *Journal of Anatomy* 228 (2): 324–37. https://doi.org/10.1111/joa.12308.

Graven, Stanley N., and Joy V. Browne. 2008. "Auditory Development in the Fetus and Infant." *Newborn and Infant Nursing Reviews* 8 (4): 187–93. https://doi.org/10.1053/j.nainr.2008.10.010.

Litovsky, Ruth. 2015. "Development of the Auditory System." In *Handbook of Clinical Neurology*, vol. 129, edited by A. J. Møller, M. F. Eggermont, A. N. Popper, and R. R. Fay. Amsterdam: Elsevier. https://doi.org/10.1016/B978-0-444-62630-1.00003-2.

White, Hunter J., Muhammad Helwany, A. R. Biknevicius, et al. 2023. "Anatomy, Head and Neck, Ear Organ of Corti." In *StatPearls* [Internet]. Treasure Island, FL: StatPearls Publishing. https://www.ncbi.nlm.nih.gov/books/NBK538335/.

Chapter 5 Reference

Bremner, A. J., and C. Spence. 2017. "The Development of Tactile Perception." In *Advances in Child Development and Behavior*, vol. 52, edited by J. Benson. Cambridge, MA: Academic Press. https://doi.org/10.1016/bs.acdb.2016.12.002.

Chapter 6 References

Boyce, J. M., and G. R. Shone. 2006. "Effects of Ageing on Smell and Taste." *Postgraduate Medical Journal* 82 (966): 239–41. https://doi.org/10.1136/pgmj.2005.039453.

Menini, Anna, ed. 2009. *The Neurobiology of Olfaction*. Boca Raton, FL: CRC Press/Taylor & Francis. https://doi.org/10.1201/9781420071993.

Rinaldi, Andrea. 2007. "The Scent of Life: The Exquisite Complexity of the Sense of Smell in Animals and Humans." *EMBO Reports* 8 (7): 629–33. https://doi.org/10.1038/sj.embor.7401029.

Sarnat, Harvey B., and Laura Flores-Sarnat. 2024. "Embryology and Clinical Development of the Human Olfactory System." *Journal of Pediatric Neurology* 22 (2): 67–78. https://doi.org/10.1055/s-0042-1758471.

van der Kolk, Bessel A. 2014. *The Body Keeps the Score: Brain, Mind, and Body in the Healing of Trauma*. New York: Viking.

Xu, Lu, Wenze Li, Venkatakaushik Voleti, Dong Jing Zou, Elizabeth M. C. Hillman, and Stuart Firestein. 2020. "Widespread Receptor-Driven Modulation in Peripheral Olfactory Coding." *Science* 368 (6487): eaaz5390. https://doi.org/10.1126/science.aaz5390.

Chapter 7 References

Boyce, J. M., and G. R. Shone. 2006. "Effects of Ageing on Smell and Taste." *Postgraduate Medical Journal* 82 (966): 239–41. https://doi.org/10.1136/pgmj.2005.039453.

Leiker, Emily K., Emma Riley, Scott Barb, Sair K. Lazzaro, Laurie Compère, Carolyn Webb, Gia Canovali, and Kymberly D. Young. 2024. "Recall of Autobiographical Memories Following Odor vs Verbal Cues among Adults with Major Depressive Disorder." *JAMA Network Open* 7 (2): e2355958. https://doi.org/10.1001/jamanetworkopen.2023.55958.

Masaoka, Yuri, Haruko Sugiyama, Atsushi Katayama, Mitsuyoshi Kashiwagi, and Ikuo Homma. 2012. "Slow Breathing and Emotions Associated with Odor-Induced Autobiographical Memories." *Chemical Senses* 37 (4): 379–88. https://doi.org/10.1093/chemse/bjr120.

Matsunaga, Masahiro, Yu Bai, Kaori Yamakawa, Asako Toyama, Mitsuyoshi Kashiwagi, Kazuyuki Fukuda, Akiko Oshida, et al. 2013. "Brain-Immune Interaction Accompanying Odor-Evoked Autobiographic Memory." *PLoS ONE* 8 (8): e72523. https://doi.org/10.1371/journal.pone.0072523.

Chapter 8 References

Holst-Wolf, Jessica M., I. Ling Yeh, and Jürgen Konczak. 2016. "Development of Proprioceptive Acuity in Typically Developing Children: Normative Data on Forearm Position Sense." *Frontiers in Human Neuroscience* 10: 436. https://doi.org/10.3389/fnhum.2016.00436.

Mavrinskaya, L. F. 1968. "Development of Muscle Spindles in Man." *Neuroscience Translations* 2 (1): 45–63. https://doi.org/10.1007/BF01125444.

Proske, Uwe, and Simon C. Gandevia. 2012. "The Proprioceptive Senses: Their Roles in Signaling Body Shape, Body Position and Movement, and Muscle Force." *Physiological Reviews* 92 (4): 1651–97. https://doi.org/10.1152/physrev.00048.2011.

Ruttle, Jennifer E., Erin K. Cressman, Bernard Marius 't Hart, and Denise Y. P. Henriques. 2016. "Time Course of Reach Adaptation and Proprioceptive Recalibration during Visuomotor Learning." *PLoS ONE* 11 (10): e0163695. https://doi.org/10.1371/journal.pone.0163695.

Yang, Nan, Gordon Waddington, Roger Adams, and Jia Han. 2019. "Age-Related Changes in Proprioception of the Ankle Complex across the Lifespan." *Journal of Sport and Health Science* 8 (6): 524–32. https://doi.org/10.1016/j.jshs.2019.06.003.

Chapter 9 References

Ferrè, Elisa R., Gabriella Bottini, Gian Domenico Iannetti, and Patrick Haggard. 2013. "The Balance of Feelings: Vestibular Modulation of Bodily Sensations." *Cortex* 49 (3): 748–58. https://doi.org/10.1016/j.cortex.2012.01.012.

Huang, Yikang, Huanyu Mao, and Yan Chen. 2022. "Regeneration of Hair Cells in the Human Vestibular System." *Frontiers in Molecular Neuroscience*. https://doi.org/10.3389/fnmol.2022.854635.

O'Reilly, Robert, Chris Grindle, Emily F. Zwicky, and Thierry Morlet. 2011. "Development of the Vestibular System and Balance Function: Differential Diagnosis in the Pediatric Population." *Otolaryngologic Clinics of North America* 44 (2): 251–71. https://doi.org/10.1016/j.otc.2011.01.001.

Pires, Anna Paula Batista de Ávila, Tatiana Rocha Silva, Maíra Soares Torres, Maria Luiza Diniz, Maurício Campelo Tavares, and Denise Utsch Gonçalves. 2022. "Galvanic Vestibular Stimulation and Its Applications: A Systematic Review." *Brazilian Journal of Otorhinolaryngology* 88 (Suppl. 3): S202–S211. https://doi.org/10.1016/j.bjorl.2022.05.010.

Chapter 10 References

Barrett, Lisa Feldman, and Karen S. Quigley. 2021. "Interoception: The Secret Ingredient." *Cerebrum: The Dana Forum on Brain Science* 2021: cer-06-21. https://pmc.ncbi.nlm.nih.gov/articles/PMC8493823/.

Brewer, Rebecca, Richard Cook, and Geoffrey Bird. 2016. "Alexithymia: A General Deficit of Interoception." *Royal Society Open Science* 3 (10): 150664. https://doi.org/10.1098/rsos.150664.

References

Brown, Brené. 2010. *The Gifts of Imperfection: Let Go of Who You Think You're Supposed to Be and Embrace Who You Are*. Center City, MN: Hazelden.

Dixon, Emily, Giulia L. Poerio, Gerulf Rieger, and Megan Klabunde. 2024. "Interoceptive Awareness and Female Orgasm Frequency and Satisfaction." *Brain Sciences* 14 (12): 1256. https://doi.org/10.3390/brainsci14121256.

McBride, Hillary L. 2021. *The Wisdom of Your Body*. Grand Rapids, MI: Brazos Press.

Mehling, Wolf E., Cynthia Price, Jennifer J. Daubenmier, Mike Acree, Elizabeth Bartmess, and Anita Stewart. 2012. "The Multidimensional Assessment of Interoceptive Awareness (MAIA)." PLoS ONE 7 (11): e48230. https://doi.org/10.1371/journal.pone.0048230.

Mehling, Wolf E., Jennifer Todd, and Zev Schuman-Olivier. 2022. "Multidisciplinary Assessment of Interoceptive Awareness, Version 2 (MAIA-2)." In *Handbook of Assessment in Mindfulness Research*, edited by Nirbhay N. Singh, Shuang Lu, and Gianluca Serafini. Cham: Springer. https://doi.org/10.1007/978-3-030-77644-2_40-1.

Mehling, Wolf E., Michael Acree, Anita Stewart, Jonathan Silas, and Alexander Jones. 2018. "The Multidimensional Assessment of Interoceptive Awareness, Version 2 (MAIA-2)." PLoS ONE 13 (12): e0208034. https://doi.org/10.1371/journal.pone.0208034.

Montoya-Hurtado, Olga, Nicolás Gómez-Jaramillo, Gloria Bermúdez-Jaimes, Luis Correa-Ortiz, Sandra Cañón, Raúl Juárez-Vela, Iván Santolalla-Arnedo, et al. 2023. "Psychometric Properties of the Multidimensional Assessment of Interoceptive Awareness (MAIA) Questionnaire in Colombian University Students." *Journal of Clinical Medicine* 12 (8): 2937. https://doi.org/10.3390/jcm12082937.

Murphy, Jennifer, Rebecca Brewer, Caroline Catmur, and Geoffrey Bird. 2017. "Interoception and Psychopathology: A Developmental Neuroscience Perspective." *Developmental Cognitive Neuroscience* 24 (April): 45–54. https://doi.org/10.1016/j.dcn.2016.12.006.

Quadt, Lisa, Hugo D. Critchley, and Sarah N. Garfinkel. 2018. "Interoception and Emotion: Shared Mechanisms and Clinical Implications." In *The Interoceptive Mind: From Homeostasis to Awareness*, edited by Manos Tsakiris and Helena De Preester, 308–25. Oxford: Oxford University Press.

Quigley, Karen S., Scott Kanoski, Warren M. Grill, Lisa Feldman Barrett, and Manos Tsakiris. 2021. "Functions of Interoception: From Energy Regulation to Experience of the Self." *Trends in Neurosciences* 44 (1): 29–38. https://doi.org/10.1016/j.tins.2020.09.008.

Schmitt, Carolyn M., and Sarah A. Schoen. 2022. "Interoception: A Multi-Sensory Foundation of Participation in Daily Life." *Frontiers in Neuroscience* 16: 875200. https://doi.org/10.3389/fnins.2022.875200.

Sun, Weiyi, Daisuke Ueno, and Jin Narumoto. 2022. "Brain Neural Underpinnings of Interoception and Decision-Making in Alzheimer's Disease: A Narrative Review." *Frontiers in Neuroscience* 16: 946136. https://doi.org/10.3389/fnins.2022.946136.

Tsakiris, Manos, and Hugo Critchley. 2016. "Interoception beyond Homeostasis: Affect, Cognition and Mental Health." *Philosophical Transactions of the Royal Society B: Biological Sciences* 371 (1708): 20160002. https://doi.org/10.1098/rstb.2016.0002.

Chapter 11 References

Diamond, David M., Adam M. Campbell, Collin R. Park, Joshua Halonen, and Phillip R. Zoladz. 2007. "The Temporal Dynamics Model of Emotional Memory

Processing: A Synthesis on the Neurobiological Basis of Stress-Induced Amnesia, Flashbulb and Traumatic Memories, and the Yerkes–Dodson Law." *Neural Plasticity* 2007: 60803. https://doi.org/10.1155/2007/60803.

Dunne, Julie, Michael Flores, Richa Gawande, and Zev Schuman-Olivier. 2021. "Losing Trust in Body Sensations: Interoceptive Awareness and Depression Symptom Severity among Primary Care Patients." *Journal of Affective Disorders* 282: 1–7. https://doi.org/10.1016/j.jad.2020.12.092.

Duquette, Patrice. 2017. "Increasing Our Insular World View: Interoception and Psychopathology for Psychotherapists." *Frontiers in Neuroscience* 11: 135. https://doi.org/10.3389/fnins.2017.00135.

Khalsa, Sahib S., Ralph Adolphs, Oliver G. Cameron, Hugo D. Critchley, Paul W. Davenport, Justin S. Feinstein, Jamie D. Feusner, et al. 2018. "Interoception and Mental Health: A Roadmap." *Biological Psychiatry: Cognitive Neuroscience and Neuroimaging* 3 (6): 501–13. https://doi.org/10.1016/j.bpsc.2017.12.004.

Sevcikova, Marcela, Marta M. Maslej, Jiri Stipl, Paul W. Andrews, Martin Pastrnak, Gabriela Vechetova, Magda Bartoskova, and Marek Preiss. 2020. "Testing the Analytical Rumination Hypothesis: Exploring the Longitudinal Effects of Problem Solving Analysis on Depression." *Frontiers in Psychology* 11 (July): 1344. https://doi.org/10.3389/fpsyg.2020.01344.

Suzuki, Naho, and Tetsuya Yamamoto. 2023. "The Influence of Interoceptive Accuracy on the Verbalization of Emotions." *Scientific Reports* 13 (1): 23210. https://doi.org/10.1038/s41598-023-49313-9.

Yerkes, Robert M., and John D. Dodson. 1908. "The Relation of Strength of Stimulus to Rapidity of Habit-Formation." *Journal of Comparative Neurology and Psychology* 18 (5): 459–82. https://doi.org/10.1002/cne.920180503.

Chapter 12 References

Atkinson, L., B. Jamieson, J. Khoury, J. Ludmer, and A. Gonzalez. 2016. "Stress Physiology in Infancy and Early Childhood: Cortisol Flexibility, Attunement and Coordination." *Journal of Neuroendocrinology* 28 (8): e12408. https://doi.org/10.1111/jne.12408.

Atzil, Shir, Wei Gao, Isaac Fradkin, and Lisa Feldman Barrett. 2018. "Growing a Social Brain." *Nature Human Behaviour* 2 (9): 624–36. https://doi.org/10.1038/s41562-018-0384-6.

Brown, Brené. 2012. *Daring Greatly: How the Courage to Be Vulnerable Transforms the Way We Live, Love, Parent, and Lead.* New York: Gotham Books.

Chan, Aldrich, and Daniel J. Siegel. 2018. "Play and the Default Mode Network: Interpersonal Neurobiology, Self, and Creativity." In *Play and Creativity in Psychotherapy*, edited by Terry Marks-Tarlow, Marion Solomon, and Daniel J. Siegel, 39–63. New York: W. W. Norton & Company.

Delgado, Mauricio R., Dominic S. Fareri, and Luke J. Chang. 2023. "Characterizing the Mechanisms of Social Connection." *Neuron* 111 (22): 3569–89. https://doi.org/10.1016/j.neuron.2023.09.012.

Dunbar, Robin. 2021. Friends: *Understanding the Power of Our Most Important Relationships*. New York: Little, Brown Spark.

Ekas, Naomi V., John D. Haltigan, and Daniel S. Messinger. 2013. "The Dynamic Still-Face Effect: Do Infants Decrease Bidding over Time When Parents Are Not Responsive?" *Developmental Psychology* 49 (6): 1027–35. https://doi.org/10.1037/a0029330.

Feldman, Ruth. 2007. "Parent-Infant Synchrony and the Construction of Shared Timing: Physiological Precursors, Developmental Outcomes, and Risk Conditions."

References

Journal of Child Psychology and Psychiatry and Allied Disciplines 48 (3–4): 329–54. https://doi.org/10.1111/j.1469-7610.2006.01701.x.

Feldman, Ruth, Romi Magori-Cohen, Giora Galili, Magi Singer, and Yoram Louzoun. 2011. "Mother and Infant Coordinate Heart Rhythms through Episodes of Interaction Synchrony." *Infant Behavior and Development* 34 (4): 569–77. https://doi.org/10.1016/j.infbeh.2011.06.008.

Hibel, Leah C., Douglas A. Granger, Clancy Blair, and Eric D. Finegood. 2015. "Maternal-Child Adrenocortical Attunement in Early Childhood: Continuity and Change." *Developmental Psychobiology* 57 (1): 83–95. https://doi.org/10.1002/dev.21266.

Kleckner, Ian R., Jiahe Zhang, Alexandra Touroutoglou, Lorena Chanes, Chenjie Xia, W. Kyle Simmons, Karen S. Quigley, Bradford C. Dickerson, and Lisa Feldman Barrett. 2017. "Evidence for a Large-Scale Brain System Supporting Allostasis and Interoception in Humans." *Nature Human Behaviour* 1 (5): 0069. https://doi.org/10.1038/s41562-017-0069.

Krzeczkowski, John E., Louis A. Schmidt, Mark A. Ferro, and Ryan J. van Lieshout. 2022. "Follow the Leader: Maternal Transmission of Physiological Regulatory Support to Distressed Infants in Real Time." *Journal of Psychopathology and Clinical Science* 131 (5): 503–13. https://doi.org/10.1037/abn0000760.

Mather, Mara, and Julian F. Thayer. 2018. "How Heart Rate Variability Affects Emotion Regulation Brain Networks." *Current Opinion in Behavioral Sciences* 19: 98–104. https://doi.org/10.1016/j.cobeha.2017.12.017.

Montirosso, Rosario, Erica Casini, Livio Provenzi, Samuel P. Putnam, Francesco Morandi, Claudia Fedeli, and Renato Borgatti. 2015. "A Categorical Approach to Infants' Individual Differences during the Still-Face Paradigm." *Infant Behavior and Development* 38 (1): 67–76. https://doi.org/10.1016/j.infbeh.2014.12.015.

Nadel, Jacqueline, Sabine Croué, Marie Jeanne Mattlinger, Pierre Canet, C. Hudelot, C. Lécuyer, and Mary Martini. 2000. "Do Children with Autism Have Expectancies about the Social Behaviour of Unfamiliar People? A Pilot Study Using the Still-Face Paradigm." *Autism* 4 (2): 133–45. https://doi.org/10.1177/1362361300004002003.

Ostlund, Brendan D., Jeffrey R. Measelle, Heidemarie K. Laurent, Elisabeth Conradt, and Jennifer C. Ablow. 2017. "Shaping Emotion Regulation: Attunement, Symptomatology, and Stress Recovery within Mother–Infant Dyads." *Developmental Psychobiology* 59 (1): 123–34. https://doi.org/10.1002/dev.21448.

Purvis, Karyn B., David R. Cross, and Wendy Lyons Sunshine. 2007. *The Connected Child: Bring Hope and Healing to Your Adoptive Family*. New York: McGraw-Hill.

Qiu, Nana, Chuangao Tang, Mengyao Zhai, Wanqing Huang, Jiao Weng, Chunyan Li, Xiang Xiao, et al. 2020. "Application of the Still-Face Paradigm in Early Screening for High-Risk Autism Spectrum Disorder in Infants and Toddlers." *Frontiers in Pediatrics* 8: 290. https://doi.org/10.3389/fped.2020.00290.

Thomas Yeo, B. T., Fenna M. Krienen, Jorge Sepulcre, Mert R. Sabuncu, Danial Lashkari, Marisa Hollinshead, Joshua L. Roffman, et al. 2011. "The Organization of the Human Cerebral Cortex Estimated by Intrinsic Functional Connectivity." *Journal of Neurophysiology* 106 (3): 1125–65. https://doi.org/10.1152/jn.00338.2011.

Tronick, Edward, Heidelise Als, Lauren Adamson, Susan Wise, and T. Berry Brazelton. 1978. "The Infant's Response to Entrapment between Contradictory Messages in Face-to-Face Interaction." *Journal of the American Academy of Child Psychiatry* 17 (1): 1–13. https://doi.org/10.1016/S0002-7138(09)62273-1.

Webb, Jonice. 2013. *Running on Empty: Overcome Your Childhood Emotional Neglect*. Morgan James Publishing.

Weinberg, M. Katherine, Marjorie Beeghly, Karen L. Olson, and Ed Tronick. 2008. "A Still-Face Paradigm for Young Children: 2½-Year-Olds' Reactions to Maternal Unavailability during the Still-Face." *The Journal of Developmental Processes* 3 (1): 44–56.

Chapter 13 References

Ayres, A. Jean. 2005. *Sensory Integration and the Child: Understanding Hidden Sensory Challenges*. 25th anniversary ed. Los Angeles: Western Psychological Services.

Bestbier, Lana, and Tim I. Williams. 2017. "The Immediate Effects of Deep Pressure on Young People with Autism and Severe Intellectual Difficulties: Demonstrating Individual Differences." *Occupational Therapy International* 2017: 7534972. https://doi.org/10.1155/2017/7534972.

Bundy, Anita C., and Shelly J. Lane, eds. 2020. *Sensory Integration: Theory and Practice*. 3rd ed. Philadelphia: F. A. Davis Company.

Kuypers, Leah M. 2011. *The Zones of Regulation: A Curriculum Designed to Foster Self-Regulation and Emotional Control*. Santa Clara, CA: Think Social Publishing, Inc.

Kranowitz, Carol Stock. 2022. *The Out-of-Sync Child: Recognizing and Coping with Sensory Processing Differences*. 3rd ed. New York: A Skylight Press/Perigee.

Mahler, Kelly. 2015. *Interoception: The Eighth Sensory System*. Kelly Mahler.

Miller, Lucy Jane. 2014. *Sensational Kids: Hope and Help for Children with Sensory Processing Disorder*. Revised ed. New York: Penguin Publishing Group.

Miller, Lucy Jane, and Doreit S. Bialer. 2011. *No Longer a Secret: Unique Common Sense Strategies for Children with Sensory or Motor Challenges*. Colorado Springs: Sensory Resources.

Mucklow, Nancy. 2009. *The Sensory Team Handbook: A Hands-On Tool to Help Young People Make Sense of Their Senses and Take Charge of Their Sensory Processing*. Kingston, ON: Michael Grass House.

Reynolds, Stacey, Shelly J. Lane, and Brian Mullen. 2015. "Effects of Deep Pressure Stimulation on Physiological Arousal." *American Journal of Occupational Therapy* 69 (3): 6903350010p1–8. https://doi.org/10.5014/ajot.2015.015560.

Schaaf, Roseann C., and Zoe Mailloux, eds. 2015. *Clinician's Guide for Implementing Ayres Sensory Integration®: Promoting Participation for Children with Autism*. Bethesda, MD: American Occupational Therapy Association. https://library.aota.org/Clinicians_Guide_for_Implementing_Ayres_SI/.

Smith Roley, Susanne, Erna I. Blanche, and Roseann C. Schaaf, eds. 2007. *Understanding the Nature of Sensory Integration with Diverse Populations*. Austin, TX: Pro-Ed.

Williams, Mary Sue, and Sherry Shellenberger. 1996. *How Does Your Engine Run?® A Leader's Guide to the Alert Program® for Self-Regulation*. Albuquerque, NM: TherapyWorks, Inc.

Winter, Leoni, Qiyin Huang, Jacquelyn V. L. Sertic, and Jürgen Konczak. 2022. "The Effectiveness of Proprioceptive Training for Improving Motor Performance and Motor Dysfunction: A Systematic Review." *Frontiers in Rehabilitation Sciences* 3: 830166. https://doi.org/10.3389/fresc.2022.830166.

References

Chapter 14 References

Chan, Aldrich, and Daniel J. Siegel. 2018. "Play and the Default Mode Network: Interpersonal Neurobiology, Self, and Creativity." In *Play and Creativity in Psychotherapy*, edited by Terry Marks-Tarlow, Marion Solomon, and Daniel J. Siegel, 39–63. Norton Series on Interpersonal Neurobiology. New York: W. W. Norton & Company.

Cinteza, Mircea. 2024. "The Six Pillars." *Mædica* 19 (2): 209–10. https://doi.org/10.26574/maedica.2024.19.2.209.

Cotman, Carl W., Nicole C. Berchtold, and Lori Ann Christie. 2007. "Exercise Builds Brain Health: Key Roles of Growth Factor Cascades and Inflammation." *Trends in Neurosciences* 30 (9): 464–72. https://doi.org/10.1016/j.tins.2007.06.011.

Davis, Catherine L., Phillip D. Tomporowski, Jennifer E. McDowell, Benjamin P. Austin, Patricia H. Miller, Nathan E. Yanasak, Jerry D. Allison, and Jack A. Naglieri. 2011. "Exercise Improves Executive Function and Achievement and Alters Brain Activation in Overweight Children: A Randomized Controlled Trial." *Health Psychology* 30 (1): 91–98. https://doi.org/10.1037/a0021766.

Delgado, Mauricio R., Dominic S. Fareri, and Luke J. Chang. 2023. "Characterizing the Mechanisms of Social Connection." *Neuron* 111 (22): 3641–59. https://doi.org/10.1016/j.neuron.2023.09.012.

Dias, Leandro, and Isabelle Menezes. 2023. "The Role of Oxytocin in Social Bonding and Its Potential Therapeutic Applications in Autism." *Revista de Psiquiatria Clínica* 50 (6): 247–56. https://doi.org/10.15761/0101-60830000000721.

Donelli, Davide, Davide Lazzeroni, Matteo Rizzato, and Michele Antonelli. 2023. "Silence and Its Effects on the Autonomic Nervous System: A Systematic Review." In *Progress in Brain Research*, vol. 280, 93–122. Amsterdam: Elsevier. https://doi.org/10.1016/bs.pbr.2023.08.001.

Dustman, R. E., R. Y. Emmerson, R. O. Ruhling, D. E. Shearer, L. A. Steinhaus, S. C. Johnson, H. W. Bonekat, and J. W. Shigeoka. 1990. "Age and Fitness Effects on EEG, ERPs, Visual Sensitivity, and Cognition." *Neurobiology of Aging* 11 (3): 193–200. https://doi.org/10.1016/0197-4580(90)90545-b.

Eisenberger, Naomi, and Matthew Lieberman. 2005. "Why It Hurts to Be Left Out: The Neurocognitive Overlap between Physical and Social Pain." In *The Social Outcast: Ostracism, Social Exclusion, Rejection, and Bullying*, edited by Kipling D. Williams, Joseph P. Forgas, and William von Hippel, 109–27. New York: Psychology Press. https://doi.org/10.4324/9780203942888-14.

Elmholdt, Else Marie, Joshua Skewes, Martin Dietz, Arne Møller, Martin S. Jensen, Andreas Roepstorff, Katja Wiech, and Troels S. Jensen. 2017. "Reduced Pain Sensation and Reduced BOLD Signal in Parietofrontal Networks during Religious Prayer." *Frontiers in Human Neuroscience* 11: 337. https://doi.org/10.3389/fnhum.2017.00337.

Fouquier, Jennifer, Nancy Moreno Huizar, Jody Donnelly, Cody Glickman, Dae-Wook Kang, Juan Maldonado, Rachel A. Jones, et al. 2021. "The Gut Microbiome in Autism: Study-Site Effects and Longitudinal Analysis of Behavior Change." *mSystems* 6 (2): e00848-20. https://doi.org/10.1128/mSystems.00848-20.

Galanter, Marc, Zoran Josipovic, Helen Dermatis, Jochen Weber, and Mary Alice Millard. 2017. "An Initial fMRI Study on Neural Correlates of Prayer in Members of Alcoholics Anonymous." *American Journal of Drug and Alcohol Abuse* 43 (1): 55–60. https://doi.org/10.3109/00952990.2016.1141912.

Gallen, Courtney L., Joaquin A. Anguera, Michael R. Gerdes, Adam J. Simon, Eva Cañadas, and Elysa J. Marco. 2021. "Enhancing Neural Markers of Attention in Children with ADHD Using a Digital Therapeutic." PLoS ONE 16 (12): e0261981. https://doi.org/10.1371/journal.pone.0261981.

References

Giri, Suman, Gopal Lamichhane, Dipendra Khadka, and Hari Prasad Devkota. 2024. "Microplastics Contamination in Food Products: Occurrence, Analytical Techniques, and Potential Impacts on Human Health." *Current Research in Biotechnology* 7 (January): 100190. https://doi.org/10.1016/j.crbiot.2024.100190.

Gómez-Pinilla, Fernando, Zhe Ying, Roland R. Roy, Raffaella Molteni, and V. Reggie Edgerton. 2002. "Voluntary Exercise Induces a BDNF-Mediated Mechanism That Promotes Neuroplasticity." *Journal of Neurophysiology* 88 (5): 2187–95. https://doi.org/10.1152/jn.00152.2002.

Grandner, Michael A., and Allan I. Pack. 2011. "Sleep Disorders, Public Health, and Public Safety." JAMA 306 (23): 2616–17. https://doi.org/10.1001/jama.2011.1833.

Gray, Peter. 2011. "The Decline of Play and the Rise of Psychopathology in Children and Adolescents." *American Journal of Play* 3 (4): 443–63.

Herring, Matthew P., Timothy W. Puetz, Patrick J. O'Connor, and Rodney K. Dishman. 2012. "Effect of Exercise Training on Depressive Symptoms among Patients with a Chronic Illness: A Systematic Review and Meta-Analysis of Randomized Controlled Trials." *Archives of Internal Medicine* 172 (2): 101–11. https://doi.org/10.1001/archinternmed.2011.696.

Holt-Lunstad, Julianne, Timothy B. Smith, and J. Bradley Layton. 2010. "Social Relationships and Mortality Risk: A Meta-Analytic Review." *PLoS Medicine* 7 (7): e1000316. https://doi.org/10.1371/journal.pmed.1000316.

Kandel, Sean. 2019. "An Evidence-Based Look at the Effects of Diet on Health." *Cureus* 11 (5): e4715. https://doi.org/10.7759/cureus.4715.

Kestly, Theresa A. 2014. *The Interpersonal Neurobiology of Play: Brain-Building Interventions for Emotional Well-Being*. 1st ed. Norton Series on Interpersonal Neurobiology. New York: W. W. Norton & Company.

Kim, M. Justin, and Sunhae Sul. 2023. "On the Relationship between the Social Brain, Social Connectedness, and Wellbeing." *Frontiers in Psychiatry* 14: 1112438. https://doi.org/10.3389/fpsyt.2023.1112438.

Kobylewski, Sarah, and Michael F. Jacobson. 2012. "Toxicology of Food Dyes." *International Journal of Occupational and Environmental Health* 18 (3): 220–46. https://doi.org/10.1179/1077352512Z.00000000034.

Komori, Teruhisa. 2018. "The Relaxation Effect of Prolonged Expiratory Breathing." *Mental Illness* 10 (1): 7669. https://doi.org/10.4081/mi.2018.7669.

Konopka, Lukasz M. 2015. "How Exercise Influences the Brain: A Neuroscience Perspective." *Croatian Medical Journal* 56 (2): 169–71. https://doi.org/10.3325/cmj.2015.56.169.

Krause, Adam J., Aric A. Prather, Tor D. Wager, Martin A. Lindquist, and Matthew P. Walker. 2019. "The Pain of Sleep Loss: A Brain Characterization in Humans." *Journal of Neuroscience* 39 (12): 2231–40. https://doi.org/10.1523/jneurosci.2408-18.2018.

Krause, Adam J., Eti ben Simon, Bryce A. Mander, Stephanie M. Greer, Jared M. Saletin, Andrea N. Goldstein-Piekarski, and Matthew P. Walker. 2017. "The Sleep-Deprived Human Brain." *Nature Reviews Neuroscience*. https://doi.org/10.1038/nrn.2017.55.

Leong, Ruth L. F., and Michael W. L. Chee. 2023. "Understanding the Need for Sleep to Improve Cognition." *Annual Review of Psychology* 74: 27–57. https://doi.org/10.1146/annurev-psych-032620-034127.

Lewis, S. J., and K. W. Heaton. 1997. "Stool Form Scale as a Useful Guide to Intestinal Transit Time." *Scandinavian Journal of Gastroenterology* 32 (9): 920–924. https://doi.org/10.3109/00365529709011203.

References

Li, Wei, Lei Ma, Guang Yang, and Wen-Biao Gan. 2017. "REM Sleep Selectively Prunes and Maintains New Synapses in Development and Learning." *Nature Neuroscience* 20 (3): 427–37. https://doi.org/10.1038/nn.4479.

Lippman, David, Mariah Stump, Erica Veazey, Sley Tanigawa Guimarães, Richard Rosenfeld, John H. Kelly, Dean Ornish, and David L. Katz. 2024. "Foundations of Lifestyle Medicine and Its Evolution." *Mayo Clinic Proceedings: Innovations, Quality & Outcomes* 8 (1): 97–109. https://doi.org/10.1016/j.mayocpiqo.2023.11.004.

Luhrmann, Tanya Marie, Kara Weisman, Felicity Aulino, Joshua D. Brahinsky, John C. Dulin, Vivian A. Dzokoto, Cristine H. Legare, et al. 2021. "Sensing the Presence of Gods and Spirits across Cultures and Faiths." *Proceedings of the National Academy of Sciences of the United States of America* 118 (5): e2016649118. https://doi.org/10.1073/pnas.2016649118.

Marcon, Rebecca A. 1993. "Socioemotional versus Academic Emphasis: Impact on Kindergartners' Development and Achievement." *Early Child Development and Care* 96 (1): 81–91. https://doi.org/10.1080/0300443930960108.

Mather, Mara, and Julian F. Thayer. 2018. "How Heart Rate Variability Affects Emotion Regulation Brain Networks." *Current Opinion in Behavioral Sciences* 19: 98–104. https://doi.org/10.1016/j.cobeha.2017.12.017.

Newberg, Andrew B., and Mark R. Waldman. 2018. "A Neurotheological Approach to Spiritual Awakening." *International Journal of Transpersonal Studies* 37 (2): 119–31. https://doi.org/10.24972/ijts.2018.37.2.119.

Ozbay, Fatih, Douglas C. Johnson, Eleni Dimoulas, C. A. Morgan, Dennis Charney, and Steven Southwick. 2007. "Social Support and Resilience to Stress: From Neurobiology to Clinical Practice." *Psychiatry (Edgmont, Pa.: Township)* 4 (5): 35–40.

Palanivelu, Lalitha, You Yin Chen, Chih Ju Chang, Yao Wen Liang, Hsin Yi Tseng, Ssu Ju Li, Ching Wen Chang, and Yu Chun Lo. 2024. "Investigating Brain–Gut Microbiota Dynamics and Inflammatory Processes in an Autistic-like Rat Model Using MRI Biomarkers during Childhood and Adolescence." *NeuroImage* 302 (November): 120899. https://doi.org/10.1016/j.neuroimage.2024.120899.

Pascual, A. Beneto. 2003. "Inadequate Sleep: A Public Health Problem." *El Sueño: Una Cuestión de Salud Pública* 1 (1): 4–9.

Pollan, Michael. 2008. *In Defense of Food: An Eater's Manifesto*. New York: Penguin Press.

Porges, Stephen W. 2009. "The Polyvagal Theory: New Insights into Adaptive Reactions of the Autonomic Nervous System." *Cleveland Clinic Journal of Medicine* 76 (Suppl. 2): S86–90. https://doi.org/10.3949/ccjm.76.s2.17.

Porges, Stephen W. 2017. *The Pocket Guide to the Polyvagal Theory: The Transformative Power of Feeling Safe*. Norton Series on Interpersonal Neurobiology. New York: W. W. Norton & Company.

Porges, Stephen W. 2021. "Polyvagal Theory: A Biobehavioral Journey to Sociality." *Comprehensive Psychoneuroendocrinology* 7: 100069. https://doi.org/10.1016/j.cpnec.2021.100069.

Rappeneau, Virginie, and Fernando Castillo Díaz. 2024. "Convergence of Oxytocin and Dopamine Signalling in Neuronal Circuits: Insights into the Neurobiology of Social Interactions across Species." *Neuroscience & Biobehavioral Reviews* 161 (June): 105675. https://doi.org/10.1016/j.neubiorev.2024.105675.

Ratey, John J., and Eric Hagerman. 2013. *Spark: The Revolutionary New Science of Exercise and the Brain*. New York: Little, Brown Spark.

References

Salmon, Peter. 2001. "Effects of Physical Exercise on Anxiety, Depression, and Sensitivity to Stress: A Unifying Theory." *Clinical Psychology Review* 21 (1). https://doi.org/10.1016/S0272-7358(99)00032-X.

Samtani, Suraj, Gowsaly Mahalingam, Ben Chun Pan Lam, Darren M. Lipnicki, Maria Fernanda Lima-Costa, Sergio Luís Blay, Erico Castro-Costa, et al. 2022. "Associations between Social Connections and Cognition: A Global Collaborative Individual Participant Data Meta-Analysis." *The Lancet Healthy Longevity* 3 (11): e783–93. https://doi.org/10.1016/S2666-7568(22)00199-4.

Simão, Talita Prado, Sílvia Caldeira, and Emilia Campos de Carvalho. 2016. "The Effect of Prayer on Patients' Health: Systematic Literature Review." *Religions* 7 (1): 11. https://doi.org/10.3390/rel7010011.

Sutoo, Den'etsu, and Kayo Akiyama. 2003. "Regulation of Brain Function by Exercise." *Neurobiology of Disease* 13 (1): 1–14. https://doi.org/10.1016/S0969-9961(03)00030-5.

Tang, Yi-Yuan, Britta K. Hölzel, and Michael I. Posner. 2015. "The Neuroscience of Mindfulness Meditation." *Nature Reviews Neuroscience* 16 (4): 213–25. https://doi.org/10.1038/nrn3916.

Taylor, Dalena L. Dillman, and Naomi Joy Wheeler. 2018. "Integrating Interpersonal Neurobiology into the Play Therapy Process: Advancing Adlerian Play Therapy." In *Applications of Neuroscience: Breakthroughs in Research and Practice*, 154–73. Hershey, PA: IGI Global. https://doi.org/10.4018/978-1-5225-5478-3.ch008.

Tibon, Roni, and Kamen A. Tsvetanov. 2022. "The 'Neural Shift' of Sleep Quality and Cognitive Aging: A Resting-State MEG Study of Transient Neural Dynamics." *Frontiers in Aging Neuroscience* 13: 746236. https://doi.org/10.3389/fnagi.2021.746236.

Trivedi, Madhukar H., Tracy L. Greer, Bruce D. Grannemann, Timothy S. Church, Daniel I. Galper, Prabha Sunderajan, Stephen R. Wisniewski, et al. 2006. "TREAD: Treatment with Exercise Augmentation for Depression: Study Rationale and Design." *Clinical Trials* 3 (3): 291–305. https://doi.org/10.1191/1740774506cn151°a.

Walker, Adam. 2024. "Sleep and Its Impact on Brain Function: A Neuroscientific Perspective." *Neuroscience and Psychiatry: Open* Access 7 (6): 287–89. https://doi.org/10.47532/npoa.2024.7(6).287-289.

Wang, Sam, and Sandra Aamodt. 2012. "Play, Stress, and the Learning Brain." *Cerebrum: The Dana Forum on Brain Science* 2012: 2.

Westphal, Andrew J., Siliang Wang, and Jesse Rissman. 2017. "Episodic Memory Retrieval Benefits from a Less Modular Brain Network Organization." *Journal of Neuroscience* 37 (13): 3523–31. https://doi.org/10.1523/jneurosci.2509-16.2017.

Wheeler, Naomi, and Dalena Dillman Taylor. 2016. "Integrating Interpersonal Neurobiology with Play Therapy." *International Journal of Play Therapy* 25 (1): 24–34. https://doi.org/10.1037/pla0000018.

Wong, Giselle C., Johanna M. Montgomery, and Michael W. Taylor. 2021. "The Gut-Microbiota-Brain Axis in Autism Spectrum Disorder." In *Autism Spectrum Disorders*, 95–113. Brisbane, Australia: Exon Publications. https://doi.org/10.36255/exonpublications.autismspectrumdisorders.2021.gutmicrobiota.

Worley, Susan L. 2018. "The Extraordinary Importance of Sleep: The Detrimental Effects of Inadequate Sleep on Health and Public Safety Drive an Explosion of Sleep Research." P & T 43 (12): 758–63. https://doi.org/10.1001/jama.2011.1833.

Xiong, Ruo-Gu, Jiahui Li, Jin Cheng, Dan-Dan Zhou, Si-Xia Wu, Si-Yu Huang, Adila Saimaiti, Zhi-Jun Yang, Ren-You Gan, and Hua-Bin Li. 2023. "The Role of Gut Microbiota in Anxiety, Depression, and Other Mental Disorders as Well as the

Protective Effects of Dietary Components." *Nutrients* 15 (14): 3258. https://doi.org/10.3390/nu15143258.

Young, Simon N. 2007. "How to Increase Serotonin in the Human Brain without Drugs." *Journal of Psychiatry & Neuroscience* 32 (6): 394–99. https://doi.org/10.1001/jama.2011.1833.

Yang, Jing, and Ping Li. 2012. "Brain Networks of Explicit and Implicit Learning." PLoS ONE 7 (8): e42993. https://doi.org/10.1371/journal.pone.0042993.

Zhang, Yu-Jie, Sha Li, Ren-You Gan, Tong Zhou, Dong-Ping Xu, and Hua-Bin Li. 2015. "Impacts of Gut Bacteria on Human Health and Diseases." *International Journal of Molecular Sciences* 16 (4): 7493–519. https://doi.org/10.3390/ijms16047493.

Zhu, Beika, Andi Wangzhou, Diankun Yu, Tao Li, Rachael Schmidt, Stacy L. De Florencio, Lauren Chao, Zeina Msheik, Yonatan Perez, Lea T. Grinberg, Salvatore Spina, Richard M. Ransohoff, Arnold R. Kriegstein, William W. Seeley, Tomasz Nowakowski, and Xianhua Piao. 2025. "G-protein-coupled Receptor ADGRG1 Drives a Protective Microglial State in Alzheimer's Disease through MYC Activation." *Neuron* 113 (19): 3224–3242.e7. https://doi.org/10.1016/j.neuron.2025.06.020. Cell+2piaolab.org+2

Chapter 15 References

Avolio, Bruce J., and William L. Gardner. 2005. "Authentic Leadership Development: Getting to the Root of Positive Forms of Leadership." *Leadership Quarterly* 16 (3): 315–38. https://doi.org/10.1016/j.leaqua.2005.03.001.

Barrett, Lisa Feldman. 2017. *How Emotions Are Made: The Secret Life of the Brain.* Boston: Houghton Mifflin Harcourt.

Brown, Brené. 2017. *Braving the Wilderness: The Quest for True Belonging and the Courage to Stand Alone*. New York: Random House.

Michie, Susan, and Janaki Gooty. 2005. "Values, Emotions, and Authenticity: Will the Real Leader Please Stand Up?" *Leadership Quarterly* 16 (3): 441–57. https://doi.org/10.1016/j.leaqua.2005.03.006.

Nagoski, Emily, and Amelia Nagoski. 2020. *Burnout: The Secret to Unlocking the Stress Cycle*. New York: Random House Publishing Group.

Narvaez, Darcia, Jaak Panksepp, Allan N. Schore, and Tracy R. Gleason, eds. 2013. *Evolution, Early Experience, and Human Development: From Research to Practice and Policy*. New York: Oxford University Press. https://doi.org/10.1093/acprof:oso/9780199755059.001.0001.

Schimmack, Ulrich, and Shigehiro Oishi. 2005. "The Influence of Chronically and Temporarily Accessible Information on Life Satisfaction Judgments." *Journal of Personality and Social Psychology* 89 (3): 395–406. https://doi.org/10.1037/0022-3514.89.3.395.

Schwartz, Shalom H. 1992. "Universals in the Content and Structure of Values: Theoretical Advances and Empirical Tests in 20 Countries." In *Advances in Experimental Social Psychology*, vol. 25, 1–65. San Diego, CA: Academic Press. https://doi.org/10.1016/s0065-2601(08)60281-6.

Sheldon, Kennon M., and Andrew J. Elliot. 1999. "Goal Striving, Need Satisfaction, and Longitudinal Well-Being: The Self-Concordance Model." *Journal of Personality and Social Psychology* 76 (3): 482–97. https://doi.org/10.1037/0022-3514.76.3.482.

References

Chapter 16 References

Barrett, Lisa Feldman. 2017. "The Theory of Constructed Emotion: An Active Inference Account of Interoception and Categorization." *Social Cognitive and Affective Neuroscience* 12 (1): 1–23. https://doi.org/10.1093/scan/nsw154.

Barrett, Lisa Feldman. 2022. "Context Reconsidered: Complex Signal Ensembles, Relational Meaning, and Population Thinking in Psychological Science." *American Psychologist* 77 (8): 1039–52. https://doi.org/10.1037/amp0001054.

Barrett, Lisa Feldman, Ralph Adolphs, Stacy Marsella, Aleix M. Martinez, and Seth D. Pollak. 2019. "Emotional Expressions Reconsidered: Challenges to Inferring Emotion from Human Facial Movements." *Psychological Science in the Public Interest* 20 (1): 1–68. https://doi.org/10.1177/1529100619832930.

Brown, Brené. 2012. *Daring Greatly: How the Courage to Be Vulnerable Transforms the Way We Live, Love, Parent, and Lead.* New York: Gotham Books.

Brown, Brené. 2017. *Braving the Wilderness: The Quest for True Belonging and the Courage to Stand Alone.* New York: Random House.

Brown, Brené. 2018. *Dare to Lead: Brave Work. Tough Conversations.* Whole Hearts. New York: Random House.

Brown, Brené. 2021. *Atlas of the Heart: Mapping Meaningful Connection and the Language of Human Experience.* New York: Random House.

Gómez-Baya, Diego, and Ramón Mendoza. 2018. "Trait Emotional Intelligence as a Predictor of Adaptive Responses to Positive and Negative Affect during Adolescence." *Frontiers in Psychology* 9: 2525. https://doi.org/10.3389/fpsyg.2018.02525.

Hambrick, Erin P., Thomas W. Brawner, and Bruce D. Perry. 2019. "Timing of Early-Life Stress and the Development of Brain-Related Capacities." *Frontiers in Behavioral Neuroscience* 13: 183. https://doi.org/10.3389/fnbeh.2019.00183.

Hill, Phyllis, and Glenn Hill. 2022. *The Connection Codes*. 3rd ed. Printopya.

Jeong, Woorim, Chun Kee Chung, and June Sic Kim. 2015. "Episodic Memory in Aspects of Large-Scale Brain Networks." *Frontiers in Human Neuroscience* 9: 454. https://doi.org/10.3389/fnhum.2015.00454.

Kim, Hongkeun. 2019. "Neural Correlates of Explicit and Implicit Memory at Encoding and Retrieval: A Unified Framework and Meta-Analysis of Functional Neuroimaging Studies." *Biological Psychology* 145: 107–20. https://doi.org/10.1016/j.biopsycho.2019.04.006.

McBride, Hillary L. 2024. *Practices for Embodied Living*. Grand Rapids, MI: Brazos Press.

McNally, Melanie. 2023. *The Emotionally Intelligent Teen: Skills to Help You Deal with What You Feel, Build Stronger Relationships, and Boost Self-Confidence*. Oakland, CA: New Harbinger Publications.

Perry, Bruce D. 1999. "The Memories of States: How the Brain Stores and Retrieves Traumatic Experience." In *Splintered Reflections: Images of the Body in Trauma*, edited by J. Goodwin and R. Attias, 9–38. New York: Basic Books.

Salovey, Peter, Laura R. Stroud, Alison Woolery, and Elissa S. Epel. 2002. "Perceived Emotional Intelligence, Stress Reactivity, and Symptom Reports: Further Explorations Using the Trait Meta-Mood Scale." *Psychology and Health* 17 (5): 611–27. https://doi.org/10.1080/08870440290025812.

Siegel, Erika H., Molly K. Sands, Wim Van den Noortgate, Paul Condon, Yale Chang, Jennifer Dy, Karen S. Quigley, and Lisa Feldman Barrett. 2018. "Emotion

References

Fingerprints or Emotion Populations? A Meta-Analytic Investigation of Autonomic Features of Emotion Categories." *Psychological Bulletin* 144 (4): 343–93. https://doi.org/10.1037/bul0000128.

Sofer, Oren Jay. 2018. *Say What You Mean: A Mindful Approach to Nonviolent Communication*. Boulder, CO: Shambhala.

Steinkrauss, Ashley C., and Scott D. Slotnick. 2024. "Is Implicit Memory Associated with the Hippocampus?" *Cognitive Neuroscience* 15 (2): 111–26. https://doi.org/10.1080/17588928.2024.2315816.

Wipfler, Patty. 2016. *Listen: Five Simple Tools to Meet Your Everyday Parenting Challenges*. Palo Alto, CA: Hand in Hand Parenting.

Appendix Reference

Thomas Yeo, B. T., Fenna M. Krienen, Jorge Sepulcre, Mert R. Sabuncu, Danial Lashkari, Marisa Hollinshead, Joshua L. Roffman, et al. 2011. "The Organization of the Human Cerebral Cortex Estimated by Intrinsic Functional Connectivity." *Journal of Neurophysiology* 106 (3): 1125–65. https://doi.org/10.1152/jn.00338.2011.

General References Cited Throughout

Berkowitz, Aaron L. 2022. "Overview of the Anatomy of the Nervous System." In *Clinical Neurology and Neuroanatomy: A Localization-Based Approach*, 2nd ed. New York: McGraw-Hill Education.

Dharani, Krishnagopal. 2015. "Functional Anatomy of the Brain." In *The Biology of Thought*, 1–21. San Diego, CA: Elsevier. https://doi.org/10.1016/b978-0-12-800900-0.00001-4.

Marzvanyan, Anna, and Ali F. Alhawaj. 2019. "Physiology, Sensory Receptors." *StatPearls* [Internet]. Treasure Island, FL: StatPearls Publishing; updated August 14, 2023. https://www.ncbi.nlm.nih.gov/books/NBK539861/.

Polin, Richard A., William W. Fox, and Steven H. Abman, eds. 2011. *Fetal and Neonatal Physiology*. 5th ed. Philadelphia, PA: Elsevier Saunders.

Rea, Paul. 2015. "Introduction to the Nervous System." In *Essential Clinical Anatomy of the Nervous System*, 1–16. San Diego, CA: Academic Press. https://doi.org/10.1016/b978-0-12-802030-2.00001-7.

www.ingramcontent.com/pod-product-compliance
Lightning Source LLC
Chambersburg PA
CBHW062130020426
42335CB00013B/1166

* 9 7 8 1 9 6 3 3 6 7 5 4 6 *